# ACUPUNCTURE PROTOCOLS FOR 300 HEALTH CONDITIONS

# ACUPUNCTURE PROTOCOLS for 300 Health Conditions

WOOSEN UR

# ACUPUNCTURE PROTOCOLS FOR 300 HEALTH CONDITIONS

*: Classical acupuncture prescriptions for clinical treatments*

Author : Woosen Ur

© 2023 Woosen Ur. All rights reserved. No part of this publication may be reproduced, distributed, or transmitted in any form or by any means, including photocopying, recording, or other electronic or mechanical methods, without the prior written permission of the publisher, except in the case of brief quotations embodied in critical reviews and certain other noncommercial uses permitted by copyright law.

The first edition in 2023

Publisher : TAI LING TERAPIAS ORIENTAIS

ISBN : 978-65-00-85836-5

# CATALOGING RECORDS

Dados Internacionais de Catalogação na Publicação ( CIP )
( Câmara Brasileira do Livro, SP, Brasil )

Ur, Woosen
Acupuncture protocols for 300 health conditions : classical acupuncture prescriptions for clinical treatments / Woosen Ur ; [ ilustração e tradução do autor ]. – Curitiba, PR : Ed. Do Autor, 2025.
Título original : Protocolos de acupuntura para 300 condições de saúde.
ISBN 978-65-00-85836-5

1. Acupuntura 2. Acupuntura – Pontos 3. Doenças –Prevenção 2. 4. Medicina chinesa tradicional 5. Medicina chinesa – Terapêutica 6. Terapia alternativa

I.Título.

25-250290

CDD-615.892
NLM-WB-369

Ídices para catálogo sistemático : Acupuntura : Medicina tradicional chinesa
615.892

Eliete Marques da Silva – Bibliotecária – CRB-8/9380

Copyright © 2023 by Woosen Ur
All rights reserved. No part of this book may be reproduced in any manner whatsoever without written permission except in the case of brief quotations embodied in critical articles and reviews.
First Printing, 2023

# DEDICATION

To dedicated healers who bridge the past and future through their hands, hearts, and minds.

To my teachers, mentors, and patients - each of you has shaped my understanding of acupuncture's profound potential.

And to those seeking knowledge within these pages, may this book serve as a guide in your journey to healing and wholeness.

# ABOUT THE AUTHOR

Woosen Ur, Ph.D.
Instagram : @woosenur
Woosen Ur was born in South Korea and has been teaching oriental medicine and therapy since 2007 in various countries and schools. He conducts research on human consciousness and traditional therapy. He conducts research on ancient classical texts of Oriental medicine, specifically focusing on therapy and human consciousness.

< Education > :
Ph.D. in Korean Medicine, Wonkwang University, South Korea
MSc in Natural Health, South Korea
BMed in Traditional Chinese Medicine, Beijing University of Chinese Medicine and Pharmacology, China
BSc in Astronomy, Seoul National University, South Korea

< Websites >:
English: https://greenaura.escolatai.com
Portuguese: https://tai-ead.escolatai.com

# DISCLAIMER

The information provided in this book is for general informational and educational purposes only, based on traditional Chinese medicine and acupuncture theories.

This book does not provide medical advice, diagnosis, treatment, or disease prevention and should not be used as a substitute for professional medical consultation. It does not guarantee specific therapeutic outcomes or endorse any medical practices. Individuals with severe health conditions should seek medical consultation.

If you have any health concerns, you should seek advice from a licensed healthcare professional before considering any treatment.

All acupuncture procedures should only be performed by properly trained and certified professionals. The determination of acupuncture prescriptions should be based on the knowledge and experience of the acupuncturist, and it is not mandatory to follow the prescriptions in this book absolutely.

All practitioners performing acupuncture must be aware of and comply with the acupuncture laws of the country in which they reside. Any improper application or use by unqualified individuals may result in unexpected risks or adverse effects, for which the author and publisher assume no responsibility.

The author and publisher shall not be held legally responsible for any consequences arising from the misuse of the information in this book or from acupuncture treatments performed by unqualified individuals.

# CONTENTS

*Dedication* ix
*About the Author* xi
*Disclaimer* xiii

| | | |
|---|---|---|
| 1 | **Preface** | 1 |
| 2 | **About this book** | 3 |
| 3 | **How to use the prescriptions, abbreviations** | 5 |
| 4 | **Courses** | 8 |
| 5 | **Principles of Acupuncture prescription in TCM** | 9 |
| 6 | **TCM disease names and Western medical disease name** | 16 |
| 7 | **Brain, mind and consciousness** | 19 |
| 8 | **Dental problems** | 43 |
| 9 | **Skin problems** | 46 |
| 10 | **Stomach, intestine, anus, digestion** | 50 |
| 11 | **Ear, nose and throat ( ENT )** | 74 |

| 12 | Eyes | 90 |
| 13 | Infection, fever | 100 |
| 14 | Women's health | 107 |
| 15 | Headache | 123 |
| 16 | Heart | 128 |
| 17 | Internal problems | 133 |
| 18 | Liver and gall bladder | 169 |
| 19 | Men's health | 174 |
| 20 | Nerve problems | 182 |
| 21 | Pediatric health issues | 190 |
| 22 | Respiratory system | 202 |
| 23 | Articulation, Bi syndrome, Muscle weakness etc | 211 |
| 24 | Kidneys and urination | 247 |
| 25 | Discussion about acupuncture for cancer | 259 |
| 26 | Bibliography | 262 |
| 27 | INDEX | 264 |

# | 1 |

# Preface

This book represents a journey into the ancient art of acupuncture, a time-tested and ever-evolving approach to holistic healing. The pages ahead are a testament to our dedication to making the profound wisdom of acupuncture accessible to all who seek it. Whether you are an experienced practitioner seeking to broaden your skills or a recent graduate from acupuncture school, this book will serve as a reference book.

This book aims to explore the relationship between traditional and contemporary approaches, providing insights into the historical and theoretical foundations of acupuncture. The information presented here is intended for educational purposes only and should not be interpreted as medical advice or a substitute for professional healthcare.

Acupuncture, as discussed in these chapters, has been traditionally practiced alongside various medical systems, and its role in integrative health continues to be an area of study and discussion. Readers are encouraged to consult a qualified healthcare professional for any medical concerns.

As you embark on this exploration, we encourage you to embrace the power of acupuncture as a complementary healing art. This book is a reference, and an invitation to uncover the transformative potential of acupuncture. Join us in discovering how this ancient practice can bring balance and vitality to your life and the lives of those you touch.

Thank you for embarking on this enlightening journey through the world of acupuncture protocols. Your quest for acupuncture commences here, and we are honored to accompany you on this path.

Yongin, South Korea, October, 2023
Woosen Ur, Ph.D.

| 2 |

# About this book

In the ever-evolving world of healthcare, acupuncture stands as a beacon of holistic medicine, offering a unique and time-tested approach to wellness. Practitioners of this ancient art, we tread a path illuminated by centuries of knowledge and wisdom. However, as we embrace the advancements of modern medicine, it becomes increasingly vital to bridge the gap between traditional acupuncture practices and the language of Western medicine. It is within this context that "Acupuncture Protocols for 300 Health Conditions " comes to life.

This book is not a proclamation of mastery; rather, it is a humble endeavor to address the needs of acupuncturists navigating the complex landscape of contemporary healthcare. Our intention is not to replace traditional TCM (Traditional Chinese Medicine) terminology or principles but to supplement and complement them. We believe that preserving the essence of TCM while integrating the language and methodology of Western medicine is the key to future therapy.

"You may ask, 'Why do acupuncturists need this book?' The answer lies in its practicality and relevance. This book enables you to seamlessly integrate Western diagnostic information into your TCM studies, deepening your understanding."

The inclusion of Western medical disease names serves a crucial purpose. It enables acupuncturists to communicate effectively with their peers in the Western medical community, facilitating collaboration and a more comprehensive approach to patient care. In an era where integrative medicine is gaining prominence, the ability to speak both languages—TCM and Western medicine—is an invaluable asset.

However, we emphasize that our embrace of Western medical terminology does not signify a departure from the rich traditions of TCM. Alongside Western disease names, we have to retain TCM disease names and syndromes. This dual approach allows you to maintain the essence of TCM while seamlessly navigating the Western medical landscape.

Navigating this book is straightforward: begin with the contents, where diseases are organized into categories. Once you've identified the category, you can easily locate the disease by its corresponding index number. Each entry provides a comprehensive acupuncture protocols based on TCM ensuring a holistic approach.

The future of acupuncture and Traditional Chinese Medicine lies in the synergy between Eastern and Western medical paradigms. We offer this book as a reference, a tool to empower acupuncturists to navigate the evolving landscape of healthcare with competence. May this book serve as a bridge between ancient wisdom and modern understanding, ultimately leading to a brighter future for our beloved field of acupuncture.

| 3 |

# How to use the prescriptions, abbreviations

This book can serve as a reference tool. To locate the protocols, you must initially ensure that you have the name of the ailment. Within the book, disease names encompass both official medical terms and simpler symptom names. In cases where a disease may not be widely recognized by its official name, the book opts for more commonly understood symptom names. This results in a varied approach, with some diseases referred to by their familiar names, while others adhere to their official designations. Then, in the table of contents at the beginning of the book, locate the group of diseases to which that disease belongs. Within the identified group of diseases, you can search for the disease alphabetically by its name. However, as some diseases may not clearly fall into a single disease group, an index at the back of the book lists all diseases alphabetically and assigns a corresponding disease index number to each. You can also use the index to find the prescription.

Within the prescriptions presented in this book, there are two categories of acupuncture points: main points and accompanying points. Main points refer to the acupoints of greater importance or those most closely related to the diseases being treated. Accompanying points, on the other hand, are acupoints of lesser significance, and their inclusion or omission is flexible. It is not mandatory to utilize all the acupoints provided in the prescription, as an excessive number of acupoints is generally not advisable.

It's important to emphasize that the prescriptions within this book are intended solely for educational and historical reference, based on traditional Chinese medicine and acupuncture theories. It does not provide medical advice, diagnosis, treatment, or prevention of any disease. Readers should consult a qualified healthcare professional before making any health-related decisions. Acupuncture procedures must be performed only by practitioners who have received proper acupuncture training and hold the necessary legal qualifications.

The selection of acupoints should be determined by a qualified acupuncturist based on a diagnosis in accordance with Traditional Chinese Medicine (TCM), taking into account the prescriptions outlined in this book as well as their own TCM knowledge and expertise. Seeking medical consultation is essential for all severe cases.

This book primarily focuses on classical Acupuncture prescriptions and doesn't delve into the prescriptions of other acupuncture systems, such as Master Tung style acupuncture, cranial acupuncture, hand therapy, abdominal acupuncture, and more, even though these systems also have their own unique functions.

In this book, abbreviated terms are employed for the names of channels and vessels as follows.
Liv : Liver channel
GB : Gall bladder channel
Ht : Heart channel
SI : Small intestine channel
SP : Spleen channel
ST : Stomach channel

Lu : Lung channel
LI : Large intestine channel
K : Kidneys channel
BL : Urinary bladder channel
PC : Pericardium channel
TB : Triple burner ( San jiao ) channel
GV : Governing vessel ( Du mai )
CV : Conception vessel ( Ren mai )
Ex : Extra acupoint ( Qi xue )

# | 4 |

# Courses

We are excited to provide an exclusive opportunity to all readers of this book. At our online platform, we offer a range of advanced oriental therapies and alternative therapies courses designed to enhance your knowledge.

To access this special offer, simply visit our course website

Websites are as follows :

Green Aura Academy :
https://greenaura.escolatai.com.
TAI LING ( Portuguese ) :
https://tai-ead.escolatai.com

We look forward to supporting your journey toward a healthier and more balanced life.

# | 5 |

# Principles of Acupuncture prescription in TCM

## (1) Characteristics

Acupuncture is a fundamental component of Traditional Chinese Medicine (TCM), dating back over two millennia. It involves the insertion of thin needles into specific acupuncture points to stimulate the body's Qi (vital energy) and restore the balance of Yin and Yang. The principles of acupuncture prescription in TCM are rooted in the ancient philosophy and theories that underpin this holistic healing system. Here are the main principles of acupuncture prescription.

**Balancing Yin and Yang:**
The core principle of TCM acupuncture is to restore the balance between Yin and Yang within the body. Yin represents the cooling, nourishing, and passive aspects, while Yang embodies warmth, activity, and stimulation. Acupuncture points are chosen to either tonify (strengthen) Yin or Yang, depending on the patient's presentation.

**Identifying the Syndrome Pattern:**

TCM diagnosis begins with identifying the specific syndrome pattern afflicting the patient. This pattern reflects the underlying imbalance in Qi, Blood, Yin, or Yang. Understanding the syndrome pattern is crucial in determining which acupuncture points to use. For example, if a patient presents with Qi deficiency, acupuncture points that tonify Qi will be selected.

### Selecting the Appropriate Acupuncture Points:

Acupuncture points are carefully chosen based on the identified syndrome pattern and the principles of meridian theory. Each acupuncture point has specific actions and indications, and their selection is based on their ability to harmonize Qi, regulate Blood, tonify Yin or Yang, and resolve stagnation or accumulation.

### Customizing Treatment for the Individual:

TCM emphasizes individualized care. Acupuncture prescriptions are tailored to the unique constitution, symptoms, and underlying imbalances of each patient. Practitioners consider factors such as the patient's age, gender, lifestyle, and overall health when selecting acupuncture points.

### Addressing Root and Branch:

TCM treatment aims not only to alleviate symptoms (branch) but also to address the root cause of the imbalance (root). Acupuncture prescriptions often include a combination of points to treat both the immediate complaints and the underlying disharmony. For example, if a patient presents with headaches (branch), the underlying Liver Qi stagnation (root) may also be addressed.

### Using Local and Distal Points:

Acupuncture points can be categorized as local (near the affected area) or distal (away from the affected area). TCM practitioners often use a combination of both local and distal points in acupuncture prescriptions. This allows for a more comprehensive approach, as stimulating distant points can influence the flow of Qi and Blood to the affected area.

**Considering Seasonal and Environmental Factors:**
TCM recognizes the influence of seasonal and environmental factors on health. Acupuncture prescriptions may be adjusted according to the patient's constitution and the prevailing season. For instance, in winter, there may be a focus on tonifying Yang and warming the body.

**Monitoring Progress and Adjusting Treatment:**
TCM acupuncture is not a one-size-fits-all approach. The progress of each patient is carefully monitored, and treatment plans are adjusted as needed. The patient's response to acupuncture, changes in symptoms, and improvements in overall well-being guide these adjustments.

**Promoting Holistic Health:**
TCM practitioners aim to promote holistic health and well-being. Acupuncture prescriptions may not only target specific complaints but also address emotional and mental aspects. The goal is to harmonize the physical, emotional, and spiritual aspects of the individual.

The principles of acupuncture prescription in TCM are deeply rooted in the ancient philosophy and theories of balance and harmony. The art and science of acupuncture involve a comprehensive assessment of the patient's condition, a thorough understanding of TCM theory, and the skillful selection of acupuncture points to restore equilibrium and facilitate the body's innate healing abilities.

## (2) TCM syndromes and acupuncture prescriptions

Traditional Chinese Medicine (TCM) recognizes a wide range of syndrome patterns, each with its own set of symptoms and corresponding acupuncture prescriptions. Although this book provides prescriptions, they should be adjusted based on your TCM diagnosis. You can add or modify the prescriptions through your diagnosis of syndromes or patterns. Below is a comprehensive list of common TCM syndromes, their typical symptoms, and acupuncture points for each syndrome.

**Qi Deficiency Syndrome:**
Symptoms : Fatigue, weakness, shortness of breath, pale complexion, low voice, spontaneous sweating, and a weak pulse.
Acupuncture Prescription:
CV-6 (Qi hai): Tonifies Qi.
ST-36 (Zu san li): Strengthens the Spleen and boosts Qi.
Lu-9 (Tai yuan): Benefits the Lung Qi.

**Yin Deficiency Syndrome:**
Symptoms: Dryness, hot flashes, night sweats, restlessness, a rapid, thin pulse, and a red tongue with little coating.
Acupuncture Prescription:
K-3 (Tai xi): Nourishes Kidneys Yin.
Ht-7 (Shen men): Calms the Heart and nourishes Yin.
SP-6 (San yin jiao): Nourishes Yin and harmonizes the Spleen.

**Yang Deficiency Syndrome:**
Symptoms: Cold extremities, fatigue, low libido, loose stools, a deep, weak pulse, and a pale, swollen tongue with teeth marks.
Acupuncture Prescription:
K-3 (Tai xi): Tonifies Kidneys Yang.
ST-36 (Zu san li): Warms and strengthens Yang.
BL-23 (Shen shu): Tonifies Kidneys Yang.

**Blood Deficiency Syndrome:**

Symptoms: Pale complexion, dizziness, blurred vision, palpitations, dry skin and hair, and a thin, weak pulse.
Acupuncture Prescription:
CV-4 (Guan yuan): Nourishes Blood.
SP-10 (Xue hai): Invigorates Blood.
Ht-7 (Shen men): Calms the Heart and nourishes Blood.

**Qi Stagnation Syndrome:**
Symptoms: Distending pain, irritability, chest tightness, sighing, a wiry pulse, and a purple tongue with possible distended sublingual veins.
Acupuncture Prescription:
Liv-3 (Tai chong): Moves Liver Qi.
PC-6 (Nei guan): Relieves chest tightness.
ST-25 (Tian shu): Regulates Qi in the abdomen.

**Blood Stagnation Syndrome:**
Symptoms: Fixed, sharp pain, dark complexion, clots in menstrual blood, ecchymosis, a choppy pulse, and a purplish tongue with possible petechiae.
Acupuncture Prescription:
SP-10 (Xue hai): Invigorates Blood.
Liv-3 (Tai chong): Moves Liver Qi and Blood.
CV-17 (Shan zhong): Promotes circulation of Qi and Blood in the chest.

**Phlegm Accumulation Syndrome:**
Symptoms: Cough with abundant white or yellow sputum, chest congestion, dizziness, a slippery pulse, and a swollen tongue with sticky coating.
Acupuncture Prescription:
CV-22 (Tian tu): Clears Phlegm from the throat.
Lu-5 (Chi ze): Expels Phlegm from the Lungs.
ST-40 (Feng long): Resolves Phlegm in the Stomach.

### Dampness Accumulation Syndrome:

Symptoms: Heavy sensation, swelling, diarrhea, a soggy pulse, and a pale, swollen tongue with sticky coating.

Acupuncture Prescription:

SP-9 (Yin ling quan): Drains Dampness from the Lower Jiao.

ST-36 (Zu san li): Strengthens the Spleen to resolve Dampness.

BL-20 (Pi shu): Regulates the Spleen and removes Dampness.

### Damp Heat Syndrome:

Symptoms: Yellow, sticky discharge, burning sensation, foul-smelling stools, a rapid, slippery pulse, and a red tongue with a greasy, yellow coating.

Acupuncture Prescription:

LI-11 (Qu chi): Clears Heat and detoxifies.

SP-9 (Yin ling quan): Resolves Dampness and Heat.

GB-34 (Yang ling quan): Clears Damp Heat from the Gallbladder.

### Blood Heat Syndrome:

Symptoms: High fever, irritability, red face, restlessness, bleeding disorders, a rapid, wiry pulse, and a red tongue with yellow coating.

Acupuncture Prescription:

Ht-8 (Shao fu): Cools Blood and reduces Heat.

LI-11 (Qu chi): Clears Heat and cools Blood.

Liv-2 (Xing jian): Clears Liver Heat.

### Accumulation of Water Syndrome:

Symptoms: Edema, bloating, heaviness, a deep, slow pulse, and a pale, swollen tongue with teeth marks.

Acupuncture Prescription:

SP-9 (Yin ling quan): Resolves Dampness and Water.

BL-22 (San jiao shu): Promotes urination and reduces edema.

K-7 (Fu liu): Regulates Water metabolism.

**Exterior Syndrome:**

Symptoms: Fever, aversion to cold, headache, body aches, a floating pulse, and a white tongue coating.

Acupuncture Prescription:

GV-14 (Da zhui): Releases the Exterior and disperses Wind.

Lu-7 (Lie que): Releases Wind and promotes sweating.

BL-12 (Feng men): Releases Wind from the back.

**Interior Heat Syndrome:**

Symptoms: High fever, irritability, red tongue with yellow coating, thirst, and a rapid pulse.

Acupuncture Prescription:

LI-11 (Qu chi): Clears Heat.

Ht-8 (Shao fu): Cools Blood and Heart Heat.

Liv-2 (Xing jian): Clears Liver Heat.

These TCM syndrome patterns and acupuncture prescriptions serve as a foundational guide for TCM practitioners in diagnosing and treating various health conditions while addressing the underlying imbalances in the body's vital substances and energy. It's important to note that TCM practices are highly individualized, and practitioners may adapt these prescriptions based on the specific needs of each patient.

# | 6 |

# TCM disease names and Western medical disease name

Here we talk about the relationship between TCM disease names and western medical disease names. Traditional Chinese Medicine (TCM) and Western medicine are two distinct healthcare systems with differing approaches to understanding and diagnosing diseases. While TCM has its own unique set of disease names and diagnostic patterns, there is often an overlap or correspondence between TCM disease names and Western medical disease names. This relationship between the two systems can be both similar and different, and understanding these relationships is essential for providing effective healthcare that integrates TCM and Western medicine principles. There are similarities between TCM and Western Medical Disease Names:

**Symptom-Based Naming:**
Both TCM and Western medicine often name diseases based on their characteristic symptoms or clinical manifestations. For example, in TCM, "Liver Qi Stagnation" describes a pattern with symptoms like irritability, chest tightness, and emotional stress, which may correspond to conditions like anxiety or non-specific chest pain in Western medicine.

**Organ-Related Diseases:**

TCM often attributes disease patterns to imbalances in specific organs, such as the Liver, Kidneys, Heart, or Spleen. Western medicine also recognizes diseases that primarily affect these organs, although the terminology and diagnostic criteria may differ. For instance, TCM's "Kidneys Yin Deficiency" may relate to Western medicine's "chronic kidneys disease."

There are differences between TCM and Western Medical Disease Names:

**Etiological Differences:**

TCM considers the root causes of disease patterns to be imbalances in Qi, Blood, Yin, Yang, and external factors like Wind, Cold, Heat, or Dampness. In contrast, Western medicine often identifies diseases based on their etiology, such as infections (e.g., bacterial or viral), genetic factors, or lifestyle-related conditions (e.g., hypertension).

**Holistic vs. Reductionist Approach:**

TCM views diseases holistically, considering the interconnectedness of various body systems and the overall balance of Qi and Blood. Western medicine often takes a reductionist approach, focusing on specific pathological mechanisms and organ dysfunction.

Integrating TCM and Western medicine can be beneficial for patient care, especially in cases where TCM can complement Western medical treatments or provide holistic support.

Here's how Western medical disease names can be used for TCM practices:

**Dual Diagnosis:**

A patient may receive both a Western medical diagnosis and a TCM diagnosis. For example, a patient with "Type 2 Diabetes" in

Western medicine may also be diagnosed with "Spleen Qi Deficiency" in TCM. The treatment plan can then address both conditions.

**Complementary Therapies:**
TCM therapies such as acupuncture, herbal medicine, dietary recommendations, and lifestyle modifications can complement Western medical treatments.

**Management of Chronic Conditions:**
For chronic conditions like hypertension, combining TCM approaches, such as acupuncture, herbal formulas, and dietary changes, can support Western medical interventions in managing symptoms.

**Patient Education:**
TCM practitioners can educate patients about the holistic principles of TCM and how they relate to Western medical diagnoses. This can empower patients to make lifestyle choices that support their overall health.

The relationship between TCM disease names and Western medical disease names reflects both similarities and differences in diagnostic approaches. Integrating TCM and Western medicine can provide a more comprehensive and personalized approach to healthcare, addressing not only the specific disease but also the overall balance and well-being of the individual patient. Collaboration between practitioners of both systems can lead to improved patient outcomes and a more holistic approach to healthcare.

# | 7 |

# Brain, mind and consciousness

### <1> Bipolar disorder, manic-depressive disorder

This is a kind of mental disease. The emotion alternates from excitement to depression or depression to excitement. Medical consultation is essential. Acupuncture treatment can be done when the patient is in depression stage. Usually phlegm blocking the orifices, liver stagnation, unstable heart of kidneys deficiency are the usual reasons in TCM way.

The main points : Si shen cong ( Ex ), GV-14 ( Da zhui ), GV-12 ( Shen zhu ), Yin tang ( Ex ), Liv-3 ( Tai chong ), PC-6 ( Nei guan ), Ht-7 ( Shen men ), GV-20 ( Bai hui ), GV-16 ( Feng fu ), GV-1 ( Chang qiang ), ST-37 ( Shang ju xu )

The accompanying points : GB-20 ( Feng chi ), BL-23 ( Shen shu ), CV-12 ( Zhong wan ), CV-6 ( Qi hai ), LI-11 ( Qu chi ), BL-10 ( Tian zhu ), Ht-8 ( Shao fu ) : reduce

The treatment principle is to open the orifices, transform the phlegm and activate the spleen, kidneys and liver. PC-6 and Ht-7 is for clearing the mind, GV-1, GV-16, GV-14 are the special points for mental disorder. The kidneys and spleen are tonified and liver is nourished for preserving the ethereal body. It is good to use moxibustion 3-5 times for the main points and use needles for the accompanying points. Si shen cong is a group of 4 points at the top of the head and at 1 cun lateral, posterior and anterior from GV-20. The soft manipulation is used on GV-16 and GB-20

### <2> Cardiac neurosis

Medical consultation is essential. The patient feels symptoms of heart like difficult breathing, oppression on chest, palpitations, nervousness, cold limbs and chest pains. Medical consultation is essential. This is a kind of neurosis. In TCM usually the weak heart is the main reason.

The main points : SP-6 ( San yin jiao ), PC-4 ( Xi men ), GV-20 ( Bai hui ), Ht-3 ( Shao hai ), Ht-6 ( Yin xi ), PC-6 ( Nei guan ), Liv-3 ( Tai chong ), BL-15 ( Xin shu ), SP-4 ( Gong sun ), ST-36 ( Zu san li )

The accompanying points : ST-40 ( Feng long ), PC-7 ( Da ling ), CV-17 ( Shan zhong ), GV-12 ( Shen zhu ), PC-8 ( Lao gong ), GV-11 ( Shen dao )

Calming the mind, regulating the heart and liver and activating the spleen are the treatment. Firstly SP-4 is needled and PC-6 is needled after that.

### <3> Cerebral anemia

The abrupt anemia in the brain is the main reason. Usually it happens with mental shock, mental stress or acupuncture treatment. The symptoms are cold sweating, nausea and vomiting, ear ringing, cold limbs, pale face, unclear vision and the patient can lose consciousness. In TCM this is usually deficiency of Qi, blood and also irregular movement of Qi.

For emergency case : If it happened because of excessive stimulation of acupuncture needle, just remove all needles. When the patient feels uncomfortable severely, strongly stimulate the point of K-1 ( Yong quan ) with wooden rod or finger, Bloodletting technique on

Shi xuan ( Ex ) or Jing well points of hands, Er jian ( Ex ). Stimulate GV-26 ( Shui gou ) or use moxibustion on GV-20 ( Bai hui ).

The main points : PC-6 ( Nei guan ), ST-36 ( Zu san li ), CV-14 ( Ju que ), GV-20 ( Bai hui ), GV-26 ( Shui gou ), CV-4 ( Guan yuan ), GV-4 ( Ming men ), CV-8 ( Shen que ) : moxibustion
The accompanying points : BL-10 ( Tian zhu ), LI-10 ( Shou san li ), CV-6 ( Qi hai ), Liv-1 ( Da dun ), SI-1 ( Shao ze )

In emergency case, usually bloodletting methods are used to open the orifices. K-1 ( Yong quan ) can be stimulated. If it is not an emergency situation and the patient easily have cerebral anemia, use GV-26 to activate the blood movement to the brain and to open orifice. Use the tonifying manipulation. The treatment principle is to open orifice, tonify Qi and blood. Shi xuan is a group of 10 points at the finger-tips. Er jian is the top of the ear.

### <4> Cerebral congestion
For some reason, the capillaries are contracted and the blood is congested in the brain. Medical consultation is essential. Usually the emotional stress or anger can be the main reason. The symptoms can be chest oppression, unclear vision, red face, palpitations, dizziness, nausea, ear ringing and headache. And in severe case, the patient can lose the consciousness.

For emergency case : Jing well points of hands or Shi xuan ( Ex ), K-1 ( Yong quan ), Er jian ( Ex ),
The main points : PC-4 ( Xi men ), K-1 ( Yong quan ), BL-10 ( Tian zhu ), GB-20 ( Feng chi ), LI-11 ( Qu chi ), Liv-3 ( Tai chong ), ST-8 ( Tou wei ), ST-36 ( Zu san li ), ST-9 ( Ren ying )
The accompanying points : SI-14 ( Jian wai shu ), CV-5 ( Shi men ), Ht-7 ( Shen men ), GB-21 ( Jian jing ), LI-4 ( He gu ), PC-6 ( Nei guan )

The emergency case is when the patient lose the consciousness. Bloodletting method is used for the emergency case points. They open the orifice and reduce the blood congestion in the brain to reduce the damage to the brain. Er jian is the top of the ear and Shi xuan is the ends of finger. The treatment principle of the main points and the accompanying points are to reduce the tension of the head and emotion, to make the patient relax, calm the mind and regulate the movement of Qi and blood. ST-9 regulate the movement of Qi and blood to reduce the blood pressure to the brain. Shi xuan is a group of 10 points at the finger-tips. The soft manipulation is used on GB-20..

### <5> CVA, brain stroke – Seven acupoints

CVA or stroke happens when the Qi movement is irregular and attacks the brain. Medical consultation is essential. Acupuncture is essential for treatment of CVA. Here is the two sets of seven acupoints which are usually considered as common prescription sets in the treatment of CVA.

Seven points for CVA (1) : GB-7 ( Qu bin ), GB-31 ( Feng shi ), ST-36 ( Zu san li ), LI-11 ( Qu chi ), GB-21 ( Jian jing ), GV-20 ( Bai hui ), GB-39 ( Xuan zhong )
Seven points for CVA (2) : GV-20 ( Bai hui ), LI-11 ( Qu chi ), ST-36 ( Zu san li ), GV-14 ( Da zhui ), GB-21 ( Jian jing ), GB-20 ( Feng chi ), PC-5 ( Jian shi )

In CVA, usually the points of head are used to activate the brain and to focus on opening the orifice to wake the consciousness up. ST-36 makes Qi descend, GB-39 is the special point for CVA. GB-39 is also the Hui meeting point of essence. GB-21 regulates the movement of Qi and used much in CVA. LI-11 cool the heat and make the Qi descend. GB-20 eliminates the wind and GV-14 activate the brain. The soft manipulation is used on GB-20.

### <6> CVA, brain stroke – aphasia

Aphasia of CVA happens when the phlegm and wind block the heart and spleen channels that pass the root of the tongue. Medical consultation is essential. The main principle of the treatment is to eliminate the phlegm and wind. Activate the heart and brain.

The main points : ST-40 ( Feng long ), SP-4 ( Gong sun ), Shang lian quan ( Ex ), GV-15 ( Ya men ), Ht-5 ( Tong li ), PC-6 ( Nei guan ), CV-22 ( Tian tu ), CV-23 ( Lian quan )
The accompanying points : GV-20 ( Bai hui ), GV-16 ( Feng fu ), LI-4 ( He gu ), K-6 ( Zhao hai ), Liv-3 ( Tai chong ), Jin jin ( Ex ), Yu ye ( Ex ), Zeng yin ( Ex )

CV-23, Shang lian quan and Zeng yin eliminate the phlegm and wind that block the tongue and make the tongue more flexible. Ht-5 activate the heart, GV-15 and GV-16 activate the brain and treat the aphasia. K-6 nourish the kidneys. Jin jin and Yu ye clear the heat in the tongue and make the tongue flexible. Bleeding method on Jin jin and Yu ye. Medium level of manipulation is used. Jin jin and Yu ye are at the blue veins under the tongue. Zeng yin is the special point to treat aphasia and it is at the lateral side of the neck, at the middle point between the adam's apple and the mandibular angle. Shang lian quan is the special point for aphasia and is at the middle point between the CV-23 and the frontal tip of the chin. The soft manipulation is used on GV-16.

### <7> CVA, brain stroke – blocking syndrome
This is an acute situation of CVA and there is sudden loss of consciousness, hands are firmly gripped and the muscles are tensed. Medical consultation is essentail. Also there are symptoms like firmly closed mouth, red face, the sound of phlegm in the throat, rough breathing or constipation etc.

The main points : PC-6 ( Nei guan ), Liv-3 ( Tai chong ), LI-4 ( He gu ), GV-16 ( Feng fu ), K-1 ( Yong quan ), Bleeding on Jing well points of hands, Liv-2 ( Xing jian ), PC-8 ( Lao gong ), GV-26 ( Shui gou ), GB-20 ( Feng chi ), GV-20 ( Bai hui ), LI-11 ( Qu chi )

The accompanying points : SP-6 ( San yin jiao ), GB-34 ( Yang ling quan ), CV-22 ( Tian tu ), ST-40 ( Feng long )

Red face, thirsty, red urine : Bleeding on Jing well points, LI-4 ( He gu ), ST-25 ( Tian shu ), LI-11 ( Qu chi ), Liv-2 ( Xing jian ), Ht-3 ( Shao hai )

Phlegm sounds in breathing : ST-40 ( Feng long ), CV-12 ( Zhong wan ), PC-6 ( Nei guan ), CV-22 ( Tian tu )

Constipation : ST-25 ( Tian shu ), ST-37 ( Shang ju xu )

Difficulty in urination : CV-3 ( Zhong ji )

Wind symptoms like convulsion, cramps at limbs, dizziness, headache : GB-20 ( Feng chi ), Liv-3 ( Tai chong ), GB-34 ( Yang ling quan ), LI-4 ( He gu ), GV-16 ( Feng fu )

The main objective of this treatment is to loosen the muscles, open the orifice, activate the brain and heart. GV-26 is to open orifice and activate the brain, Bleeding Jing well points of the hands will clear the heat in the brain and reduce the damage to the brain. GB-20 eliminate the wind, PC-8 and PC-6 will clear the heat of the heart and make the consciousness recover. Liv-2 to clear the liver heat, ST-25 and ST-37 to treat the constipation and eliminate the heat. Liv-3 to regulate the Qi of liver and CV-22 to regulate the movement of Qi. ST-40 to eliminate the phlegm. Bleeding method is used for Jing well points. Reducing manipulation is used. The soft manipulation is used on GB-20 and GV-16.

### <8> CVA, brain stroke – facial paralysis

Medical consultation is essential. There are two kinds of facial paralysis. One is from infection and the other is from CVA. This prescription is about facial paralysis from CVA. In TCM, opening the orifices and activating the facial nerves are the main treatment principle. But most of all, treating the original causes of facial paralysis is the most important. Usually through the local points of the face, eliminating the wind from the head and regulating the movement of Qi and blood are the main methods.

The main points : ST-4 ( Di cang ), GV-26 ( Shui gou ), TB-17 ( Yi feng ), ST-43 ( Xian gu ), SI-18 ( Quan liao ), LI-4 ( He gu ) on the healthy side, ST-6 ( Jia che ), ST-2 ( Si bai ), Qian zheng ( Ex ), ST-44 ( Nei ting )

The accompanying points : GB-14 ( Yang bai ), GB-20 ( Feng chi ), BL-2 ( Zan zhu ), ST-36 ( Zu san li ), SI-19 ( Ting gong ), Jia cheng jiang ( Ex ), Liv-3 ( Tai chong )

The medium level manipulation can be applied. The needles are applied on only one side of the face. You can alternatively treat the pathological side and the healthy side of the face. Jia cheng jaing is at the 1 cun lateral side of the CV-24. Qian zheng is at 0.5 ~ 1 cun anterior to the auricular lobe. Electric acupuncture can be applied. The soft manipulation is used on GB-20.

### <9> CVA, brain stroke – paralysis of lower limbs

Medical consultation is essential. Because the reason of the paralysis is from CVA, the most important thing is to treat the CVA, activating the brain to recover from CVA. There are some extra acupoints ( EX ) in this prescription. The main idea is activating the GB, ST, BL channels, the Yang channels of the lower limbs. The classical acupuncture's idea is activating the Yang channels mainly for CVA because Yang channel will move Qi and blood and can treat the paralysis and also it will eliminate the wind, the pathogen that causes CVA.

The main points : ST-40 ( Feng long ), Tan li ( Ex ), LI-4 ( He gu ), GB-34 ( Yang ling quan ), GB-41 ( Zu lin qi ), ST-38 ( Tiao kou ), GB-30 ( Huan tiao ), GB-39 ( Xuan zhong ), ST-36 ( Zu san li ), GB-31 ( Feng shi )

The accompanying points : Jiu nei fan ( Ex ), Jiu wai fan ( Ex ), ST-41 ( Jie xi ), Zhi tan 6 ( Ex ), Liv-3 ( Tai chong ), BL-60 ( Kun lun ), GV-20 ( Bai hui )

Jiu wan fan is 1 cun external from BL-57 ( Cheng shan ) and Jiu nei fan is 1 cun internal from BL-57 ( Cheng shan ). Zhi tan 6 is 0.5 cun below ST-37 ( Shang ju xu ). Tan li is 5 fingers width higher than the external side angle of knee cap. Use the long needle for ST-38 ( Tiao kou ), GB-39 ( Xuan zhong ), GB-34 ( Yang ling quan ) and K-1 ( Tai xi ) and apply the strong manipulation. Usually after the strong manipulation on the pathological side, the soft manipulation is done for the healthy side.

### <10> CVA, brain stroke – paralysis of upper limbs

Medical consultation is essential. Because the reason of the paralysis is from CVA, the most important thing is to treat the CVA, activating the brain to recover from CVA. There are some extra acupoints ( EX ) in this prescription. The main idea is activating the TB, LI, SI channels, the Yang channels of the upper limbs. The classical acupuncture's idea is activating the Yang channels mainly for CVA because Yang channel will move Qi and blood and can treat the paralysis and also it will eliminate the wind, the pathogen that causes CVA.

The main points : TB-4 ( Yang chi ), Ba xie ( Ex ), LI-4 ( He gu ), SI-3 ( Hou xi ), LI-11 ( Qu chi ), Ht-3 ( Shao hai ), TB-5 ( Wai guan ), PC-6 ( Nei guan ) : you can use the long needle to penetrate the two points with one needle.

The accompanying points : Bloodletting technique on Lu-5 ( Chi ze ), LI-10 ( Shou san li ), GB-21 ( Jian jing ), LI-14 ( Bi nao ), TB-14 ( Jian liao ), SI-6 ( Yang lao ), LI-15 ( Jian yu )

Ba xie is a group of points at the sides of the fingers. Use the long needle from SI-3 to LI-4, TB-5 to PC-6 and Li-11 to Ht-3. Strong manipulation is applied on the pathological side and after that, the soft manipulation is applied on the healthy side. The treatment method is to activating the Yang channels to treat the paralysis.

### <11> CVA, brain stroke – prevention

The prevention method of CVA is recorded in the classic of acupuncture, Zhen jiu da cheng. The idea is to direct the Qi movement to the lower area of the body for the ascending Qi not to attack the brain and to nourish the kidneys Yin to hold the floating Yang. Medical consultation is essential.

The main points : ST-36 ( Zu san li ), GB-39 ( Xuan zhong ) : from the classic of acupuncture, Zhen jiu da cheng.
The accompanying points : GV-20 ( Bai hui ), GB-20 ( Feng chi ), LI-10 ( Shou san li ), Liv-3 ( Tai chong ), SP-6 ( San yin jiao ), LI-11 ( Qu chi ), PC-6 ( Nei guan )

ST-36 and GB-39 direct the Qi to the lower part. GB-39 is also the Hui meeting point of the essence and it nourishes the essence of kidneys and liver. PC-6 opens orifice, regulates the Qi and transforms phlegm. Li-10 directs the Qi to the lower part and clears the ascending heat. GV-20 dissipates the attacking Qi on the brain. Usually use moxibustion mainly on the main points. After the application of moxibustion for 3 days, take a rest for 1 day and continue. The accompanying points are used together when the possibility of CVA is high. The soft manipulation is used on GB-20

### <12> CVA, brain stroke – prodrome ( Symptoms before CVA attacks )

The prodrome of CVA is the symptoms that usually happen before CVA attacks. The patient have cognitive impairment and motor function impairment, dizziness, headache, fatigue, speech difficulties, sensory impairment or visual problems. But some patient does not show any prodrome before CVA attack. Commonly the hypertension patients have these prodromes. The main idea of treatment is to eliminate the wind, clear the heat, regulate the Yin and Yang, open the orifice and calm the Yang of liver. Medical consultation is essential.

The main points : ST-36 ( Zu san li ), GB-39 ( Xuan zhong ), GV-20 ( Bai hui ), bleeding on the Jing well points of hands and feet, bleeding on the blue veins on the back of ear, Shi xuan ( Ex ), Qi duan ( Ex ), PC-6 ( Nei guan ), GB-20 ( Feng chi )

The accompanying points : GV-26 ( Shui gou ), LI-4 ( He gu ), GB-21 ( Jian jing ), LI-11 ( Qu chi ), Liv-3 ( Tai chong ), SP-6 ( San yin jiao )

Shi xuan is a group of points at the finger-tips. Qi duan is a group of points at the tips of toes. Bleeding method is used for Shi xuan, Jing well points, Qi duan, Veins on the back of ear. Strong manipulation is used for the other points. Medical check and treatment are urgent. The soft manipulation is used on GB-20.

### <13> CVA, brain stroke – syndrome of collapse

The patients have the symptoms of collapse like unclear consciousness, opened mouth, closed eyes, loose hands and muscles, the reddish cheeks but pale face, cold limbs and uncontrolled urine and feces. Usually this is from the deficiency of Qi and Yang. Moxibustion can be used to eliminate the coldness and tonify the Yang. Medical consultation is essential.

The main points : GV-20 ( Bai hui ), GV-26 ( Shui gou ), CV-4 ( Guan yuan ), PC-6 ( Nei guan ), GV-4 ( Ming men ), CV-6 ( Qi hai ), K-1 ( Yong quan ),

The accompanying points : CV-8 ( Shen que ) : moxibustion, LI-4 ( He gu ), PC-8 ( Lao gong ), GV-16 ( Feng fu ), GB-20 ( Feng chi ), GB-39 ( Xuan zhong ), ST-36 ( Zu san li ), GV-14 ( Da zhui ), Jing well points of hands, SP-6 ( San yin jiao )

Moxibustion is used on CV-4, CV-6, CV-8, ST-36, BL-23, GV-14 and GV-4. The extreme deficiency like collapse cases uses moxibustion instead of needles. Use less number of needles because the patients can lose Qi through needles. Urgent medical treatment is necessary. The prescription is to regulate the Yin and Yang, tonify the Yang and Qi. Open the orifice and nourish liver and kidneys. Jing well points are for the emergency situation. The soft manipulation is used on GV-16, GB-20.

### <14> Epilepsy (1)

Abruptly the patient can have convulsion and lose consciousness, have phlegm on the mouth, sometimes make the strange sounds. But there are also mild cases like only slight spasm on the mouth, hands or feet. The main cause is the liver and gall bladder wind, phlegm blocking the orifice. Transforming the phlegm, opening the orifice and calming the mind are the main treatment principles. Medical consultation is essential.

The main points : Ht-7 ( Shen men ), GV-15 ( Yan men ), GB-20 ( Feng chi ), GV-1 ( Chang qiang ), CV-15 ( Jiu wei ), SI-3 ( Hou xi ), BL-15 ( Xin shu ), PC-6 ( Nei guan ), Liv-3 ( Tai chong ), GV-14 ( Da zhui ), SP-4 ( Gong sun )

The accompanying points : CV-12 ( Zhong wan ), Yao qi ( Ex ), BL-62 ( Shen mai ), K-6 ( Zhao hai ), GV-11 ( Shen dao ), GV-20 ( Bai hui ), LI-4 ( He gu ), ST-40 ( Feng long )

Yao qi is located at the middle point between the two BL-32 and it is the special point for epilepsy. GV-15 and GV-14 open the orifice. SI-3 and K-6 nourish the kidneys, CV-15 is a special point for epilepsy. Use the strong manipulation to eliminate the phlegm and open the orifice. Soft manipulation is used on GB-20. Long needle is used for GV-1.

### <15> Epilepsy (2)

Abruptly the patient can have convulsion and lose consciousness, have phlegm on the mouth, sometimes make the strange sounds. But there are also mild cases like only slight spasm on the mouth, hands or feet. The main cause is the liver and gall bladder wind, phlegm blocking the orifice. Transforming the phlegm, opening the orifice and calming the mind are the main treatment principles. Medical consultation is essential.

The main points : CV-15 ( Jiu wei ), SP-1 ( Yin bai ), Liv-3 ( Tai chong ), GV-1 ( Chang qiang ), GV-14 ( Da zhui ), GV-12 ( Shen zhu ), Lu-11 ( Shao shang ), Yao qi ( Ex )

The accompanying points : BL-10 ( Tian zhu ), K-1 ( Yong quan ), K-6 ( Zhao hai ), BL-62 ( Shen mai ), LI-4 ( He gu ), GV-23 ( Shang xing )

These points are used for treatment of mental disorder or epilepsy. GV-23 opens the orifice and GV-1 is the special point for epilepsy. The accompanying points nourish the kidneys and regulate the brain. Yao qi is located at the middle point between the two BL-32 and it is the special point for epilepsy. The moxibustion is used on the main points and the strong needle manipulation on the accompanying points. Treat for 3 days, take a rest for 1 day and continue.

### <16> Epilepsy (3)

Abruptly the patient can have convulsion and lose consciousness, have phlegm on the mouth, sometimes make the strange sounds. But there are also mild cases like only slight spasm on the mouth, hands or feet. The main cause is the liver and gall bladder wind, phlegm blocking the orifice. Transforming the phlegm, opening the orifice and calming the mind are the main treatment principles. Medical consultation is essential.

The main points : Ht-7 ( Shen men ), CV-14 ( Ju que ), ST-40 ( Feng long ), Yao qi ( Ex ), GV-26 ( Shui gou ), GB-20 ( Feng chi ),

PC-5 ( Jian shi ), GV-14 ( Da zhui ), GV-16 ( Feng fu ), BL-62 ( Shen mai ), LI-4 ( He gu )

The accompanying points : CV-12 ( Zhong wan ), Liv-3 ( Tao chong ), SP-6 ( San yin jiao ), GB-34 ( Yang ling quan ), K-6 ( Zhao hai )

Treat everyday or once for two days. Medium level manipulation of needle. K-6 is connected with the extraordinary channel of Yin qiao mai and BL-62 is connected with the extraordinary channel of Yang qiao mai. If the attack happens at night, use the point K-6 instead of BL-62 and if the attack happens at daytime, use the point BL-62 instead of K-6. Yao qi is at the middle point between the two BL-32 and it is the special point for epilepsy. GV-16, GV-26, GV-14 open the orifice to treat the epilepsy. The liver and gall bladder channels are used to eliminate the wind. And Some points for transforming the phlegm. Yao qi is located at the middle point between the two BL-32 and it is the special point for epilepsy.

### <17> EPS ( Extrapyramidal symptoms )

This problem is usually caused by typical antipsychotic drugs that antagonize dopamine D2 receptor in brain. Medical consultation is essential. Other causes include brain damage or meningitis but EPS usually refers to medication-induced cases. Symptoms are trembling hands, shaking body, increasing tension on the face, stiff expression on the face. The main idea to treat is opening the orifice, activating the brain, calming the wind and mind.

The main points GV-4 ( Ming men ), PC-6 ( Nei guan ), GB-13 ( Ben shen ), GB-34 ( Yang ling quan ), GB-20 ( Feng chi ), GV-26 ( Shui gou ), GV-20 ( Bai hui ), ST-36 ( Zu san li ), : LI-15 ( Jian yu ), LI-10 ( Shou san li ), GB-31 ( Feng shi ), LI-11 ( Qu chi ), BL-19 ( Dan shu )

The accompanying points : GV-14 ( Da zhui ), GV-12 ( Shen zhu ), TB-5 ( Wai guan ), K-9 ( Zhu bin ), GV-8 ( Jin suo ), BL-41 ( Fu fen

), SP-6 ( San yin jiao ), LI-4 ( He gu ), GB-36 ( Wai qiu ), BL-18 ( Gan shu ), BL-23 ( Shen shu ), GB-30 ( Huan tiao ), PC-4 ( Xi men )

Points on GV, Liv and GB activate the brain and open the orifice. The points on the head activate the brain. Points on the limbs are to calm the uncontrollable movements. Medium level manipulation is used. Needle and moxibustion can be used together alternatively.

### <18> Hysteria (1)

This is a kind of neurosis, easily happens for female patients who have introvert personality and too sensitive. Medical consultation is essential. Long term mental stress, unsatisfied desires and nervousness are the main cause. The symptoms are emotional outburst, shortness of breath, anxiety, fainting, spasm, bizarre movements, deafness, seizures, blindness, loss of sensation, hallucination, being overly dramatic or excited etc. The treatment principle is opening the orifice, calm the mind, wind, clearing the heat and phlegm and liberating the liver Qi stagnation.

The main points : GV-20 ( Bai hui ), Ht-7 ( Shen men ), GV-26 ( Shui gou ), Liv-3 ( Tai chong ), Liv-14 ( Qi men ), GV-20 ( Bai hui ), PC-6 ( Nei guan ), K-1 ( Yong quan ), BL-10 ( Tian zhu )
The accompanying points : SP-4 ( Gong sun ), GV-15 ( Ya men ), CV-22 ( Tian tu ), Ht-5 ( Tong li ), Li-11 ( Qu chi ), Yin tang ( Ex ), GB-34 ( Yang ling quan ), CV-23 ( Lian quan )

Use the long needle and strong manipulation for LI-11 and GB-34. GV-26 open the orifice and clear the brain. PC-6 transforms the phlegm and calm the mind. GV-15 clears the brain. Soft manipulation is used for GV-15.

### <19> Hysteria (2)

This is a kind of neurosis, easily happens for female patients who have introvert personality and too sensitive. Medical consultation is essential. Long term mental stress, unsatisfied desires and nervousness are the main cause. The symptoms are emotional outburst, shortness of breath, anxiety, fainting, spasm, bizarre movements, deafness, seizures, blindness, loss of sensation, hallucination, being overly dramatic or excited etc. The treatment principle is opening the orifice, calm the mind, wind, clearing the heat and phlegm and liberating the liver Qi stagnation.

The main points :), PC-6 ( Nei guan ), GB-34 ( Yang ling quan ), Liv-8 ( Qu quan ), Ht-7 ( Shen men ), BL-10 ( Tian zhu ), GV-20 ( Bai hui ), Liv-3 ( Tai chong ), GB-20 ( Feng chi ), BL-18 ( Gan shu ), SP-4 ( Gong sun )

The accompanying points : PC-3 ( Qu ze ), Liv-2 ( Xing jian ), GB-41 ( Zu lin qi ), CV-17 ( Shan zhong ), CV-6 ( Qi hai ), BL-32 ( Ci liao ), BL-23 ( Shen shu ), SP-6 ( San yin jiao ), GV-12 ( Shen zhu ), CV-12 ( Zhong wan )

Change the accompanying points every time. Medium level needle manipulation. GB-20, GB-41, Liv-3, GB-34 calm the liver wind and liberate the liver Qi stagnation. BL-18 nourish the liver to hold the floating wind. Soft manipulation is used on GB-20.

**<20> Insomnia**

There are many kinds of insomnia and they all have different causes. Medical consultation is essential. If the cause is from other diseases, the treatment of those diseases has to be the primary treatment. Insomnia can happen from emotional problem, deficiency of heart and spleen, hypertension and headache, difficulty in digestion, menopause syndrome or brain bleeding etc. The prescription here is focusing on calming the mind by regulating the heart and kidneys. This can be applied to emotional, anxiety or mental nervousness too.

The main points : Ht-7 ( Shen men ), PC-6 ( Nei guan ), BL-23 ( Shen shu ), An mian ( Ex ), Yin tang ( Ex ), SP-6 ( San yin jiao ), Liv-2 ( Jing jian ), GV-20 ( Bai hui )

The accompanying points : K-1 ( Yong quan ), LI-11 ( Qu chi ), PC-5 ( Jian shi ), BL-15 ( Xin shu ), LI-4 ( He gu ), K-6 ( Zhao hai )

The main idea is to nourish the kidneys to harmonize it with the heart.. Yin tang is at the middle point between the two eyebrows and An mian is at the middle point between the TB-17 and GB-20. Soft manipulation is used for this prescription.

## <21> Neurasthenia

Excessive use of brain or long term mental stress can cause Neurasthenia. Medical consultation is essential. Chronic disease or weak constitution also can cause it. Usually the patients experience ear ringing, loss of concentration, insomnia, palpitations, dizziness, headache, anxiety, too much dreams or nervousness. Medical consultation is essential. The main idea of treatment is to calm the mind, nourish the heart and spleen, nourish the kidneys and liver and to liberate the liver.

The main points : Yin tang ( Ex ), PC-6 ( Nei guan ), GB-20 ( Feng chi ), GV-20 ( Bai hui ), An mian ( Ex ), Ht-7 ( Shen men ), Liv-3 ( Tai chong ), SP-6 ( San yin jiao ), BL-20 ( Pi shu )

The accompanying points : Ht-5 ( Tong li ), LI-4 ( He gu ), ST-36 ( Zu san li ), CV-4 ( Guan yuan ), BL-18 ( Gan shu ), BL-15 ( Xin shu ), BL-21 ( Wei shu )

An mian is at the middle point between GB-20 and TB-17. Yin tang is the middle point between the two eyebrows. GB-20 has a strong effect to calm the mind by calming the wind. It also activates the brain. CV-4, BL-18 nourish the kidneys and liver. BL-15 nourish the heart. BL-20 and BL-21 tonify spleen and stomach to nourish the whole body. If the patient thinks in excess it damages spleen and stomach. Soft needle manipulation is used for this prescription and moxibustion is used for CV-4

### <22> Neurosis – OCD, phobia, anxiety disorder

Neurosis is not psychosis or neuroticism but it has severe mental and physical symptoms like distress, OCD ( Obsessive-compulsory disorder ), dizziness, heavy head, fear ( a variety of phobia ), palpitations, nervousness, feeling unsafe, chest oppression, fear of death etc. But it does not include hallucination or delusions. Medical consultation is essential. The main cause is personal difficulty in adapting to one's environment or inability to change one's life patterns.

The main points : PC-6 ( Nei guan ), GB-34 ( Yang ling quan ), GB-20 ( Feng shi ), GV-1 ( Chang qiang ), Ht-7 ( Shen men ), Si shen cong ( Ex ), GV-20 ( Bai hui ), K-1 ( Yong quan ), Liv-3 ( Tai chong ), Liv-14 ( Qi men )

The accompanying points : GV-23 ( Shang xing ), GV-20 ( Bai hui ), BL-15 ( Xin shu ), CV-17 ( Shan zhong ), BL-23 ( Shen shu ), GV-16 ( Feng fu ), BL-10 ( Tian zhu )

Si shen cong is a group of four points 1 cun posterior, anterior and lateral from GV-20. The treatment idea is calming the mind by nourishing heart and kidneys. Opening the orifice and calming the wind. Medium level manipulation is used. Soft manipulation is used on GV-16.

### <23> Night crying of babies

This is a kind of neurosis that has the symptom of crying at night without special reason. Medical consultation is essential. The main idea of treatment is calming the mind and eliminating the heat, tonifying the kidneys and relieving the body tension.

The main points : GV-12 ( Shen zhu ), ST-36 ( Zu san li ), LI-2 ( Er jian ), CV-12 ( Zhong wan ), PC-9 ( Zhong chong ), Liv-3 ( Tai chong ), GV-4 ( Ming men ), PC-6 ( Nei guan )

The accompanying points : Both sides of vertebrae, Navel area, Area at the top of head ( this area is not used for a little baby whose fontanelles are not closed yet. ), Area of abdominal muscles,

Bleeding method on PC-9 and Moxibustion on navel area, GV-12, GV-4, LI-2. Medium level manipulation is used. Soft massage on the points can be used for relaxation. For safety reasons, do not use the area at the top of an infant's head if their fontanelles have not closed. Do not needle the belly button to avoid the risk of infection.

### <24> Parkinson's disease

The main cause is the nerve cells in the basal ganglia in brain become impaired or die. Medical consultation is essential. Because of this, the brain produces less dopamine and it causes the Parkinson's disease. The main symptoms are shaking the body, uncontrollable movement, stiffness, loss of balance, difficulty in speaking, stiff face expression. In TCM, Liver responsible for shaking. Acupuncture can not completely cures the Parkinson's disease. The main idea of treatment in acupuncture is tonifying the kidneys, liver to nourish the brain, calming the wind, activate the local channels to relieve the body shaking. The liver and gall bladder channels are important to calm the wind.

The main points : GB-20 ( Feng chi ), GB-31 ( Feng shi ), Liv-3 ( Tai chong ), BL-23 ( Shen shu ), GV-16 ( Feng fu ), GB-34 ( Yang ling quan ), GV-26 ( Shui gou ), GV-20 ( Bai hui ), CV-4 ( Guan yuan ), GB-39 ( Xuan zhong ),

The accompanying points : GV-12 ( Shen zhu ), LI-11 ( Qu chi ), BL-18 ( Gan shu ), BL-10 ( Tian zhu ), LI-4 ( He gu ), CV-12 ( Zhong wan ), BL-32 ( Ci liao ), BL:-19 ( Dan shu )

The points of the liver and gall bladder channel are used to nourish the liver and to calm the wind. Medium level of manipulation is used. Soft manipulation is used on GV-16

### <25> Schizophrenia (1)

This is a serious mental disease which has hallucinations, delusions, and extremely abnormal thinking and behavior. Medical consultation is essential. This disease easily happens in juvenile age. There are two types of Schizophrenia. One is calm type and the other is excited type. Calm type patients usually are in silence and speechless, alternate crying and laughing, severely sad, think they are extremely inferior or feel victimized. The excited type shows violence, insomnia, talk too much, excited excessively. It will be a long term treatment. The phlegm blocking the orifice, heat in heart, deficiency of kidneys, spleen or stagnation of liver are pathology. The main idea of treatment is using the GV channel that enters the brain. Stimulating GV channel opens the orifice. Many points around the head, GV, PC and Ht are used to open the orifice and clear the heat of heart. In case of excited type usually use reducing manipulation.

The main points : PC-6 ( Nei guan ), GV-16 ( Feng fu ), LI-4 ( He gu ), SI-3 ( Hou xi ), PC-8 ( Lao gong ), LI-11 ( Qu chi ), ST-37 ( Shang ju xu ), K-1 ( Yong quan ), K-3 ( Tai xi ), GV-26 ( Shui gou ), GV-14 ( Da zhui ), GV-13 ( Tao dao ), GV-12 ( Shen zhu ), ST-40 ( Feng long )

The accompanying points : PC-7 ( Da ling ), PC-5 ( Jian shi ), Liv-2 ( Xing jian ) or Liv-3 ( Tai chong ), Tai yang ( Ex ) : bloodletting technique, GB-35 ( Yang jiao ) or GB-36 ( Wai qiu ), GB-6 ( Xuan li ), Ht-7 ( Shen men ), BL-62 ( Shen mai )

GV-26, GV-15 activate the brain and open the orifice. GV-14, GV-13, GV-12 activate the brain, clear the heat. ST-40 transforms the phlegm that is blocking the orifice. K-1 also activates the brain. GB-35 is the Xi cleft point of Yang wei mai and GB-36 is the Xi cleft point of GB channel. GB-35 and GB-36 has the function to treat Schizophrenia. Strong manipulation is used. And the soft manipulation is used on GV-16

### <26> Schizophrenia (2)

This is a serious mental disease which has hallucinations, delusions, and extremely abnormal thinking and behavior. Medical consultation is essential. This disease easily happens in juvenile age. There are two types of Schizophrenia. One is calm type and the other is excited type. Calm type patients usually are in silence and speechless, alternate crying and laughing, severely sad, think they are extremely inferior or feel victimized. The excited type shows violence, insomnia, talk too much, excited excessively. It will be a long term treatment. The phlegm blocking the orifice, heat in heart, deficiency of kidneys, spleen or stagnation of liver are pathology. The main idea of treatment is using the GV channel that enters the brain. Stimulating GV channel opens the orifice. Many points around the head, GV, PC and Ht are used to open the orifice and clear the heat of heart. In case of excited type usually use reducing manipulation. Soft manipulation is used on GV-16

The main points : Hai quan ( Ex ), ST-37 ( Shang ju xu ), SI-3 ( Hou xi ), Lu-11 ( Shao shang ), GV-14 ( Da zhui ), GV-26 ( Shui gou ), PC-7 ( Da ling ), SP-1 ( Yin bai ), GV-16 ( Feng fu ), GV-23 ( Shang xing ), PC-8 ( Lao gong )

The accompanying points : CV-24 ( Cheng jiang ), K-1 ( Yong quan ), LI-11 ( Qu chi ), BL-62 ( Shen mai ), GB-35 ( Yang jiao ) or GB-36 ( Wai qiu ), ST-40 ( Feng long ), PC-6 ( Nei guan ), PC-5 ( Jian shi )

Moxibustion or needle can be used for this prescription. Long needle is used for SI-3 to needle it deeply to LI-4. Strong manipulation is used except GV-16. Hai quan clears the internal heat that causes the problem. GB-35 is the Xi cleft point of Yang wei mai and GB-36 is the Xi cleft point of GB channel. GB-35 and GB-36 has the function to treat Schizophrenia. The main idea of treatment is to clear the internal heat.

### <27> Sydenham's chorea ( SC )

This is a neurological disorder resulting from infection via Group A beta-hemolytic streptococcus (GABHS), a kind of bacterium. Medical consultation is essential. The symptoms are irregular and rapid involuntary movements of the limbs and facial muscles. The symptoms are like dancing. SC more frequently happens in girls of childhood than boys. The treatment idea is to regulate the movement of Qi and blood on the whole body. The local points are used following the symptoms.

The main points : GB-34 ( Yang ling quan ), GB-31 ( Feng shi ), GV-12 ( Shen zhu ), Liv-2 ( Xing jian ), GV-16 ( Feng fu ), GV-4 ( Ming men ), GV-20 ( Bai hui ), ST-36 ( Zu san li ), K-1 ( Yong quan ), GB-20 ( Feng chi )

The accompanying points :

Symptoms on upper limbs : Ba xie ( Ex ), Shang ba xie ( Ex ), LI-4 ( He gu ) to SI-3 ( Hou xi ), LI-11 ( Qu chi ) to Ht-3 ( Shao hai ), LI-10 ( Shou san li )

Symptoms on lower limbs : Ba feng ( Ex ), Shang ba feng ( Ex ), GB-39 ( Xuan zhong ), GB-34 ( Yang ling quan ) to SP-9 ( Yin ling quan ), ST-36 ( Zu san li )

Symptoms on face : ST-7 ( Xia guan ), TB-17 ( Yi feng ), BL-10 ( Tian zhu ),

Ba xie is a group of points at the sides of the fingers. Shang ba xie is slightly above the Ba xie on the dorsal side of hand. Ba feng is a group of points at the sides of the toes. Shang ba feng is slightly above the Ba feng. Ba xie, Shang ba xie, Ba feng and Shang ba feng can regulate the Qi and blood of the upper and lower limbs to calm the involuntary movements of the limbs. The local points on the limbs are used to regulate the Qi and blood on the limbs. Strong manipulation is used.

The soft manipulation is used on GV-16 and GB-20. The accompanying points are used at the pathological sides.

### &lt;28&gt; Writer's cramp, graphospasm

The patients experience the difficulty in writing because of muscular spasm on the forefinger and thumb. Medical consultation is essential. The clear cause is not known. The treatment idea is calming the wind, relieving the tension on hands and calming the mind.

The main points : GB-31 ( Feng shi ), LI-4 ( He gu ), GV-20 ( Bai hui ), Yin tang ( Ex ), Ht-3 ( Shao hai ), GB-34 ( Yang ling quan ), PC-6 ( Nei guan ), GV-14 ( Da zhui ), LI-11 ( Qu chi ), Liv-3 ( Tai chong ), Ht-7 ( Shen men ), GB-20 ( Feng chi )

The accompanying points : GV-16 ( Feng fu ), Liv-2 ( Xing jian ), GB-12 ( Wan gu ), SI-8 ( Xiao hai ), PC-7 ( Da ling ), Lu-5 ( Chi ze ), PC-8 ( Lao gong )

The local points on hands are used. Channels of GV and PC and used to calm the trembling. Strong manipulation is used. The soft manipulation is used on GV-16 and GB-2

### &lt;29&gt; Depression

Depression affects a person's thoughts, behavior, feelings, and well-being. Medical consultation is essential. Those who suffer from depression often lose motivation, interest, and pleasure in activities that once brought them joy. They feel deep sadness, difficulty concentrating, and changes in appetite and sleep, which can be a reaction to events such as the loss of a loved one, a symptom of physical illnesses, or a side effect of medications.

Depression can be brief or prolonged and, in severe cases, lead to suicidal thoughts. The feeling of hopelessness and discouragement makes it difficult to perform daily tasks and find pleasure in activities. In Chinese medicine, the main pathological alterations include imbalances in the flow of Qi, resulting in Qi stagnation and internal blockage by stagnant phlegm. This can lead to the liver transforming into fire due to stagnation, as well as deficiencies in the liver and spleen, and simultaneously in the heart and spleen, along with Yang deficiency in the spleen and kidneys, affecting the brain. The treatment principle aims to eliminate Qi stagnation, control liver fire, transform phlegm, and regulate organs such as the liver, spleen, heart, and kidneys, as well as open the orifices to stimulate the brain.

The main points: VG20 (Bai Hui), Si Shen Cong (Ex), Yin Tang (Ex), PC6 (Nei Guan), BP4 (Gong Sun), C7 (Shen Men), F2 (Xing Jian), IG4 (He Gu), E40 (Feng Long), F14 (Qi Men), VG26 (Shui Gou).

The accompanying points: VG26 (Shui Gou), VG16 (Feng Fu), PC7 (Da Ling), C5 (Tong Li), PC8 (Lao Gong), B15 (Xin Shu), B19 (Dan Shu), VC12 (Zhong Wan), C9 (Shao Chong), VG11 (Shen Dao).

VG20 and Si Shen Cong awaken the brain and clear consciousness. Yin Tang and VG20 make cerebral perception clearer. PC6 is also a very important point to awaken the brain and eliminate phlegm from the heart. PC6 and BP4 are used in combination to treat emotional problems or palpitations. C7 calms the mind and F2 eliminates and regulates liver fire. If the patient does not present many fire symptoms, F3 can be used instead of F2. E40 is used to transform phlegm. F14, F2, and IG4 relieve liver Qi stagnation.

The patient can breathe deeply while manipulating the needle in PC6, which will relieve Qi stagnation in the chest, allowing the patient to feel lighter both in the chest and breathing pattern (depression often causes a feeling of tightness in breathing and chest). VG26 opens the orifices to awaken the brain. VG16 is useful when the patient presents psychotic symptoms, as it also awakens the brain and clears the mind. B19 eliminates Gallbladder (GB) stagnation and can also regulate it.

The combination of the heart and pericardium channels is beneficial. Points and manipulation can be selected according to the patient's pattern diagnosis.

# | 8 |
# Dental problems

**<30> Dentoalveolar abscess**

The collected pus in the dental alveoli. Usually the gum becomes swollen, dark and red, moving teeth. Medical or dental consultation is essential. ST channel passes the upper alveole and LI channel passes the lower alveole. The treatment idea is eliminating inflammation on the location of abscess, removing abscess. The selection of points are local points, points that clear the heat and remove the inflammation.

The main points : For upper alveole, GB-20 ( Feng chi ), ST-36 ( Zu san li ) : reducing technique, ST-7 ( Xia guan ), ST-44 ( Neiting ) / For lower alveole, LI-11 ( Qu chi ), ST-6 ( Jia che ), LI-7 ( Wen liu ), and LI-4 ( He gu ) on the opposite side, ST-5 ( Da ying )

The accompanying points : GB-31 ( Feng shi ), K-3 ( Tai xi ), SP-6 ( San yin jiao ), BL-20 ( Pi shu ), ST-25 ( Tian shu ), CV-12 ( Zhong wan ), ST-37 ( Shang ju xu ) : reducing technique, K-1 ( Yong quan ), BL-21 ( Wei shu ), BL-23 ( Shen shu ), LI-2 ( Er jian )

Following the syndromes, kidneys can be tonified for deficiency of kidneys or spleen can be tonified for deficiency of spleen. If the syndrome is deficiency, usually the situation becomes chronic. ST-25 eliminates the heat from ST channel and promote intestine to remove feces. ST-44 clears the stomach heat, LI-4 clears the large intestine heat. LI-7 is the Xi cleft point of large intestine. Strong manipulation for the main points. The soft manipulation is used on GB-20. Moxibustion can be used for the accompanying points.

### <31> Gingivitis

This is an inflammation problem in gum. Medical or dental consultation is essential. The symptoms are swollen gum, pain, swollen and red cheeks, insomnia because of pain and nervousness, fatigue or fever. The main cause is mental stress that produces internal heat, that attacks the gum. The treatment idea is clearing the heat through channels of LI and ST. LI channel is more about the lower gum and ST channel is more about the upper gum.

The main points : LI-2 ( Er jian ), ST-6 ( Jia che ), Ashi points, LI-4 ( He gu ), ST-44 ( Nei ting ), ST-7 ( Xia guan ), LI-11 ( Qu chi ), ST-36 ( Zu san li ), GB-20 ( Feng chi ), PC-4 ( Xi men ), LI-7 ( Wen liu )

The accompanying points : GB-31 ( Feng shi ), TB-23 ( Si zhu kong ), TB-21 ( Er men ), CV-12 ( Zhong wan ), BL-23 ( Shen shu ), K-3 ( Tai xi ), Tai yang ( Ex )

LI and ST channels are Yang ming channel that has much Qi and blood and easily clears the heat or regulate the Qi and blood to treat the pains. Tai yang is at the temporal region of the head. Local points are used to reduce the local heat. PC-4 cool the blood and treat the acute situation. For the chronic case or deficiency, BL-23 and K-3 are used to nourish the kidneys. Bloodletting methods can be used for the regions near Ashi points.

### <32> Toothache

The toothache can have a variety of causes. Medical or dental consultation is essential. And acupuncture treatment for toothache is temporary painkilling. It is better check the dental exam to find out the causes of toothache.

The main points : ST-6 ( Jia che ), LI-2 ( Er jian ), ST-44 ( Nei ting ), K-1 ( Yong quan ), LI-4 ( He gu ), LI-11 ( Qu chi ), ST-7 ( Xia guan ), ST-36 ( Zu san li )

For chronic case or deficiency : SP-6 ( San yin jiao ), K-2 ( Ran gu ), K-3 ( Tai xi )

The accompanying points : LI-7 ( Wen liu ), TB-17 ( Yi feng ), K-3 ( Tai xi ), GB-20 ( Feng chi ), K-7 ( Fu liu ), ST-37 ( Shang ju xu )

LI channel for lower toothache and ST channel for upper toothache. The above points clear the heat on ST and LI channels and direct the heat to lower part. K-7 nourishes kidneys to strengthen the teeth. ST-6 and ST-7 are local points. LI-7 is the Xi cleft point of large intestine. GB-12 and TB-17 eliminate the wind. Strong manipulation is used. The soft manipulation or no manipulation is used on GB-20 ( follow the safety guide of acupuncture ). In case of deficiency or chronic case, nourishing kidneys is necessary. K-1 directs the fire downwards.

# | 9 |

# Skin problems

### <33> Alopecia areata ( patchy hair loss )

The symptoms are unpredictable and patchy hair loss. It is considered as an autoimmune problem. Medical consultation is essential. Sometimes, patients lose eyebrows as well. Usually the genetic and environmental factors are considered as the main causes that makes the immune system mistakenly attack the hair follicles. In TCM there are many syndromes as liver Qi stagnation ( mental stress ), deficiency of Qi and blood, Yin and Yang, fire for deficiency or excess fire etc. The prescription here is to remove the inflammation on the hair follicles, activate the Qi and blood circulation on the head, clear the heat on head. More points can be added following the result of TCM diagnosis.

The main points : LI-4 ( He gu ), GB-20 ( Feng chi ), Si shen cong ( Ex ), Liv-3 ( Tai chong ), Ashi on the head, , GV-20 ( Bai hui ), CV-4 ( Guan yuan ), BL-10 ( Tian zhu )

The accompanying points: GB-31 ( Feng shi ), BL-13 ( Fei shu ), Ht-7 ( Shen men ), GV-14 ( Da zhui ), LI-11 ( Qu chi ), K-7 ( Fu liu )

Ashi on the head activate the movement of Qi and blood on the local area. BL-13 to nourish the lung to nourish the head skin. LI-11 to clear the heat on head. Liv-3 liberate the Qi stagnation of liver.

GB-20 and GB-31 eliminate the wind in the upper body. Si shen cong is the extra acupoints on the head. That is a group of four points, at the vertex, 1 cun respectively posterior, anterior, and lateral to GV-20 ( Bai hui ). Soft stimulation on Ashi can be used by Seven stars needles. Medium level stimulation for LI-4 and Liv-3. Calming the mind is necessary.

### <34> Corn, Clavus

The symptom is thickening of the skin. The main causes are intermittent pressure and frictional forces. These result in clinical and histological hyperkeratosis.

The main and accompanying points : Ashi ( Corn )
Use moxibustion cone on the Ashi. 6 times for a day.

### <35> Hives, Urticaria

This disease can be spontaneous, inducible, acute or chronic. Medical consultation is essential. Acute one has less than 6 weeks duration and chronic one has more than 6 weeks duration. The symptoms are bumps and raised patches The patient feel itchy and look swollen. The treatment idea is to clear the heat, eliminate the wind to treat the itchy skin.

The main points : GV-14 ( Da zhui ), GB-31 ( Feng shi ), SP-8 ( Di ji ), GB-20 ( Feng chi ), SP-6 ( San yin jiao ), BL-40 ( Wei zhong ) : bloodletting technique, SP-10 ( Xue hai ) or Bai chong wo ( Ex ), LI-11 ( Qu chi ), LI-4 ( He gu )
The accompanying points : Lu-7 ( Lie gue ), BL-12 ( Feng men ), ST-37 ( Shang ju xu ), CV-12 ( Zhong wan ), Liv-2 ( Xing jian ), LI-15 ( Jian yu ), ST-25 ( Tian shu ), BL-25 ( Da chang shu )

LI-4, LI-11, GV-14 clear the heat. GB-20 eliminate the wind. SP-6 nourishes the Yin and blood. SP-10 moves blood to eliminate the wind. The strong manipulation is used for the main points except

GB-20. Bai chong wo ( Ex. ) is the special point for itchy skin. The location is at 3 cun proximal to the superior border of the patella, at a depression on the bulge of the vastus medialis muscle.

### <36> Pruritus, itching

Itching skin is the main symptoms. Medical consultation is essential. The patient can not sleep well because of itching skin. In case of old people, the dry skin can be the cause and it is related with the change of climate, menstruation or menopause. The treatment idea is to clear the heat from lung and large intestine, move blood to eliminate the wind.

The main points : BL-17 ( Ge shu ), BL-40 ( Wei zhong ), LI-4 ( He gu ), LI-11 ( Qu chi ), SP-6 ( San yin jiao ), GV-14 ( Da zhui ), Xue hai ( SP-10 ) or Bai chong wo ( Ex ), Liv-3 ( Tai chong ), GB-20 ( Feng chi )

The accompanying points : BL-15 ( Xin shu ), BL-18 ( Gan shu ), Lu-10 ( Yu ji ), Lu-5 ( Chi ze ), ST-37 ( Shang ju xu ), BL-12 ( Feng men ), LI-15 ( Jian yu ), GV-20 ( Bai hui ), GV-12 ( Shen zhu )

LI-4, LI-11, GV-14 clear the heat. GB-20 eliminate the wind. SP-10, SP-6, BL-17 move blood the eliminate the wind. GV-20 calms the mind. Medium level manipulation is used. In case of chronic case, moxibustion is used on ST-36, BL-17, GV-14, LI-11, SP-6, SP-10, GB-20. Bai chong wo ( Ex. ) is the special point for itchy skin. The location is at 3 cun proximal to the superior border of the patella, at a depression on the bulge of the vastus medialis muscle.

### <37> Warts

The symptoms are rough, skin colored bumps that form on the skin. Medical consultation is essential. Usually it is caused by HPV ( Human Papilloma Virus ) by infection. It is contagious. The treatment idea is killing the warts by heat ( moxibustion )

The main points and accompanying points : Ashi ( Warts )

Use moxibustion cone on the wart. Every time use moxibustion cone 6 times a day.

# | 10 |

# Stomach, intestine, anus, digestion

### <38> Appendicitis

The treatment of appendicitis in acupuncture is only for mild symptoms cases or chronic cases. Medical consultation is essential. If the patients have severe symptoms, high fever or risk of peritonitis, it is safe to do surgery in the hospital. The treatment idea is to eliminate the local inflammation, move Qi and blood. Mainly the ST channel that passes the area of appendix is used for treatment. The local points near appendix should not be needled too deeply because it has the risk of peritonitis.

The main points : ST-37 ( Shang ju xu ), ST-27 ( Da ju, on the right side ), Lan wei ( Ex ), LI-11 ( Qu chi ), CV-6 ( Qi hai ), SP-14 ( Fu jie, on the right side ), ST-25 ( Tian shu ), ST-40 ( Feng long )

The accompanying points : LI-10 ( Shou san li ), ST-44 ( Nei ting ), BL-24 ( Qi hai shu ), BL-25 ( Da chang shu ), LI-4 ( He gu ), GB-34 ( Yang ling quan ), ST-39 ( Xia ju xu )

The strong manipulation is used for acute case and moxibustion is used for chronic case. ST-25 is the front mu alarm point of large intestine. BL-25 is the back shu point of large intestine. ST-39 is the lower

He sea point of small intestine. Lan wei ( Ex ) is the special point for appendicitis, this point can be used for acute or chronic cases. The location of Lan wei is 2 cun below ST-36 ( Zu san li ).

### <39> Bacillary dysentery

This is a gastrointestinal disease. Medical consultation is essential. The cause is bacterial infection and the symptoms are fever, severe diarrhea, blood or pus in feces, nausea and vomiting or stomach pain. Sometimes it can be life-threatening and needs hospitalization in an intensive care unit. This disease more easily happens in summer and autumn. It is related with war and it was popular in the first and the second world war. Usually the low sanitization countries have more cases. The treatment idea is to remove the inflammation, move Qi and blood of Yang ming channels. The acute case is the syndrome of excess fire and the chronic case is the syndrome of deficiency. Following the syndrome, selection of the accompanying points can be made.

The main points : ST-37 ( Shang ju xu ), PC-6 ( Nei guan ), SP-4 ( Gong sun ), CV-12 ( Zhong wan ), LI-4 ( He gu ), ST-36 ( Zu san li ), ST-25 ( Tian shu )
The accompanying points :
For abdominal pain : Liv-3 ( Tai chong ), SP-6 ( San yin jiao ), CV-4 ( Guan yuan ), ST-34 ( Liang qiu )
For diarrhea : SP-9 ( Yin ling quan ), Zhi xie ( Ex )
For fever : LI-2 ( Er jian ), ST-44 ( Nei ting ), GV-14 ( Da zhui ) and LI-11 ( Qu chi ), Ht-8 ( Shao fu ) : reducing technique to reduce the heat

Mainly the points on the ST and LI channels are important because they treat the inflammation in the Yang ming channel. Zhi xie is an extra acupoint for diarrhea and the location is at 0.5 cun above CV-4 and it stops diarrhea. LI-11 is the He sea point of large intestine. PC-6 regulates the digestive tract. ST-37 is the lower He sea point of large intestine. ST-25 is the front mu alarm point of large intestine.

LI-2 clear the heat from large intestine. ST-34 is the Xi cleft point of stomach and it relieves the abdominal pain. CV-4 is the front mu alarm point of small intestine and it also tonifies Qi and blood. Strong manipulation is used for main points. The moxibustion can be used for chronic cases. Considering the symptoms, the prescription can be modified.

### <40> Colitis (1)

Emotional problem, mental stress, autoimmune problem or infection can be the causes. Medical consultation is essential. Patients have the symptoms like bloated abdomen, frequent diarrhea, retention of feces inside, low appetite, nausea and vomiting or fever. Treatment idea is regulating large intestine using LI and ST channels to stop diarrhea, relieving pain, eliminating inflammation, activating Qi of spleen.

The main points : ST-36 ( Zu san li ), ST-44 ( Nei ting ), CV-4 ( Guan yuan ), ST-37 ( Shang ju xu ), ST-25 ( Tian shu ), LI-11 ( Qu chi ), LI-4 ( He gu ), LI-2 ( Er jian ), BL-25 ( Da chang shu )

The accompanying points : LI-10 ( Shou san li ), SP-4 ( Gong sun ), CV-6 ( Qi hai )

For solid feces : SP-14 ( Fu jie, left side ), TB-6 ( Zhi gou )

For diarrhea : Zhi xie ( Ex )

For abdominal pain : ST-34 ( Liang qiu ), CV-12 ( Zhong wan )

Zhi xie is 0.5 cun above CV-4 and it stops diarrhea. LI-4 regulates large intestine and treat fever and infection. ST-25 is front mu alarm point of large intestine. ST-37 is lower He sea point of large intestine. LI-2, LI-10 clear the heat and inflammation from large intestine. ST-34 relieve abdominal pain and stops diarrhea. TB-6 promotes movement of large intestine. Strong manipulation is used for the main points. The moxibustion and soft manipulation is used for the chronic and deficiency cases.

### <41> Colitis (2) – acute case

Acute colitis commonly happens with old foods, alcohol, stimulating foods like spices. Medical consultation is essential. Symptoms are abdominal pain, diarrhea or blood in feces. In case of infection, the patient can have fever. The old patients and children can have the severe cases. The treatment idea is regulating the intestine by ST, LI, and SP channels, eliminating the dampness and inflammation.

The main points : ST-36 ( Zu san li ), BL-25 ( Da chang shu ), BL-20 ( Pi shu ), BL-23 ( Shen shu ), CV-12 ( Zhong wan ), ST-25 ( Tian shu ), ST-27 ( Da ju ), CV-6 ( Qi hai )

The accompanying points : LI-10 ( Shou san li ), SP-6 ( San yin jiao ), CV-4 ( Guan yuan )

For abdominal pain : ST-34 ( Liang qiu ), GB-36 ( Wai qiu ), ST-44 ( Nei ting ), Liv-3 ( Tai chong )

For coldness : GV-4 ( Ming men )

Use moxibustion : ST-36 ( Zu san li ), ST-37 ( Shang ju xu ), CV-4 ( Guan yuan ), Li nei ting ( Ex )

Li nei ting is an extra acupoint. The location is at the bottom side of ST-44 that regulates the large intestine. CV-12 is the Hui meeting point of Fu organs and front mu alarm point of stomach. ST-34 is the Xi cleft point of stomach and it regulates the stomach and intestine, stops abdominal acute pains. Strong manipulation is used for the main points. Moxibustion is used for ST-25, CV-6, CV-4, LI-11 and Li nei ting. GB-36 is used for the case of peritonitis or pain.

### <42> Colitis (3) – chronic case

There are many causes for chronic colitis. Medical consultation is essential. Chronic case happens with old patients, low immunity, allergic chronic colitis or acute case can transform into the chronic case. The symptoms are oppression or uncomfortable feelings on abdomen, diarrhea or borborygmus. Treatment idea is tonifying spleen, kidneys, Qi, blood and regulating the movement of intestine.

The main points : ST-40 ( Feng long ), ST-36 ( Zu san li ), BL-25 ( Da chang shu ), BL-23 ( Shen shu ), ST-25 ( Tian shu ), SP-4 ( Gong sun ), CV-4 ( Guan yuan ), K-16 ( Huang shu ), GV-4 ( Ming men ), BL-20 ( Pi shu ), ST-27 ( Da ju )

The accompanying points : ST-39 ( Xia ju xu ), SP-6 ( San yin jiao ), LI-10 ( Shou san li ), CV-12 ( Zhong wan ), SI-3 ( Hou xi )

For abdominal pain : ST-34 ( Liang qiu ), CV-6 ( Qi hai )

For borborygmus : CV-6 ( Qi hai ), SP-2 ( Da du )

K-16 regulates the intestine, BL-20 and BL-23 tonifies the spleen and kidneys. ST-25 is the front Mu alarm point of large intestine. ST-40 eliminate the pus from intestine, ST-39 is the lower He sea point of small intestine. Medium level manipulation is used. Moxibustion can be used for CV-4, 6, ST-25, GV-4, ST-36 in case it needs.

### <43> Constipation

Although constipation is a common symptom and not a disease but it can cause other severe diseases. Medical consultation is essential. It is necessary to treat the constipation or regulate the bowl movement to maintain the overall health. The treatment idea is promoting the bowl movement using ST and LI channel. There are excess syndrome and deficiency syndrome. Following the syndromes, the accompanying points can be modified.

The main points : ST-36 ( Zu san li ), ST-37 ( Shang ju xu ), ST-25 ( Tian shu ), SP-4 ( Gong sun ), PC-6 ( Nei guan ), SP-14 ( Fu jie, on the left side ), LI-4 ( He gu ), CV-4 ( Guan yuan ), ST-27 ( Da ju ), TB-6 ( Zhi gou )

The accompanying points : LI-11 ( Qu chi ), SP-15 ( Da heng ), Lu-7 ( Lie que ), Liv-2 ( Xing jian ), LI-2 ( Er jian ), Ht-7 ( Shen men ), LI-10 ( Shou san li ), BL-25 ( Da chang shu )

ST-25 is the front Mu alarm point of large intestine, CV-4 is the front Mu alarm point of small intestine. ST-37 is the lower He sea point of large intestine. TB-6 activates the triple burners and helps the bowl remove the feces. PC-6 regulates the stomach and directs the Qi downwards. SP-4 ( Gong sun ) is the luo connecting point of SP channel and it activates the movement of intestine. Ht-7 calm the mind. Medium level manipulation is used.

### <44> Diarrhea (1)

There are many kinds of causes. Understanding the possible causes is important. Medical consultation is essential. One of the most common and simple cause is irregular eating or old food. Diarrhea with simple causes can be easily treated in acupuncture. The treatment idea is activating Qi and blood in Yang ming channel, activating large intestine, eliminating dampness by activating spleen and relieve the pain. In case of chronic case with deficiency, tonifying spleen and kidneys yang is necessary.

The main points : SP-9 ( Yin ling quan ), CV-8 ( Shen que, moxibustion, Do not needle this point ), Zhi xie ( Ex ) or CV-4 ( Guan yuan ), ST-36 ( Zu san li ), LI-7 ( Wen liu ), LI-11 ( Qu chi ), ST-25 ( Tian shu ), ST-34 ( Liang qiu )

The accompanying points : ST-37 ( Shang ju xu ), ST-39 ( Xia ju xu )

Aggravation with mental stress : LI-4 ( He gu ), Liv-3 ( Xing jian ), Ht-7 ( Shen men ), GV-20 ( Bai hui ), Yin tang ( Ex )

ST-34 regulates the Qi and blood in stomach channel and it stops abdominal pain. Zhi xie is 0.5 cun above CV-4 and it stops diarrhea. Salt, ginger piece or aconite piece can be used for indirect moxibustion on CV-8. LI-7 is the Xi cleft point of large intestine. BL-60 is used for dawn diarrhea. CV-8 tonifies Yang of kidneys and spleen. In case of dawn diarrhea, it is necessary to tonify Kidneys Yang. Continuous moxibustion on abdomen is effective for chronic diarrhea. SP-9 strengthens spleen and eliminates the dampness. GV-20 and Ht-7 is used for mental stress that causes diarrhea.

### <45> Diarrhea (2)

There are many kinds of causes. Understanding the possible causes is important. Medical consultation is essential. One of the most common and simple cause is irregular eating or old food. Diarrhea with simple causes can be easily treated in acupuncture. The treatment idea is activating Qi and blood in Yang ming channel, activating large intestine, eliminating dampness by activating spleen and relieve the pain. In case of chronic case with deficiency, tonifying spleen and kidneys yang is necessary.

The main points : SP-15 ( Da heng ), BL-25 ( Da chang shu ), ST-34 ( Liang qiu ), ST-36 ( Zu san li ), CV-12 ( Zhong wan ), LI-11 ( Qu chi ), Zhi xie ( Ex ), ST-25 ( Tian shu ), GV-20 ( Bai hui )

The accompanying points : SP-9 ( Yin ling quan ), Liv-3 ( Tai chong ), BL-20 ( Pi shu ), K-7 ( Fu liu ), LI-10 ( Shou san li ), ST-37 ( Shang ju xu ), CV-6 ( Qi hai ), Ht-7 ( Shen men ), CV-8 ( Shen que, use moxibustion, Do not needle this point )

Zhi xie is an extra acupoints. The location is at 0.5 cun above CV-4 and it stops diarrhea. ST-34 regulates Qi and blood and stops abdominal pain. ST-25 is the front Mu alarm point of large intestine. BL-60 is used for dawn diarrhea. CV-12 is the front Mu alarm point of stomach and Hui meeting point of Fu organs. Indirect moxibustion with salt, ginger piece or aconite is used for CV-8. SP-15 eliminates dampness and activates spleen. Ht-7 and GV-20 is for diarrhea with mental stress. In case of dawn diarrhea, it is necessary to tonify Kidneys Yang. Strong manipulation is used for acute case and medium level manipulation is used for chronic case. Regular moxibustion on abdomen has a good effect.

### <46> Diarrhea (3) – with colic

There are many kinds of causes. Understanding the possible causes is important. Medical consultation is essential. One of the most common and simple cause is irregular eating or old food. Diarrhea with simple causes can be easily treated in acupuncture. The treatment idea is activating Qi and blood in Yang ming channel, activating large intestine, eliminating dampness by activating spleen and relieve the pain. In case of chronic case with deficiency, tonifying spleen and kidneys yang is necessary.

The main points : CV-12 ( Zhong wan ), ST-25 ( Tian shu ), ST-34 ( Liang qiu ), LI-11 ( Qu chi ), LI-10 ( Shou san li ), ST-36 ( Zu san li ),
The accompanying points : SP-9 ( Yin ling quan ), ST-37 ( Shang ju xu ), Zhi xie ( Ex )
For fever : GV-14 ( Da zhui ), LI-11 ( Qu chi ), LI-4 ( He gu )
For mental stress : Liv-3 ( Tai chong ), LI-4 ( He gu ), GV-20 ( Bai hui ), Yin tang ( Ex )
For nausea : PC-6 ( Nei guan ), SP-4 ( Gong sun )

Medium level manipulation is used for the main points. Zhi xie is an extra acupoint for diarrhea and the location is at 0.5 cun above CV-4 and it stops diarrhea. ST-37 is lower He sea point of large intestine. ST-25 is front mu alarm point of large intestine. SP-6 eliminate dampness. ST-34 regulates the movement of stomach and relieve the pain. Liv-3 has to be reduced to relieve the liver Qi stagnation.

### <47> Duodenal ulcer

Symptoms are abdominal pain with empty stomach on the upper right side of abdomen, vomiting blood, nausea and vomiting. Medical consultation is essential. Usually it aggravates at night. The treatment idea is regulating Qi and blood of digestive tract of stomach, large intestine to relieve the pain of duodenum. Acupuncture is only for relieving pain of duodenal ulcer.

The main points : PC-6 ( Nei guan ), Liv-3 ( Tai chong ), ST-39 ( Xia ju xu ), ST-34 ( Liang qiu ), SP-4 ( Gong sun ), LI-11 ( Qu chi ), K-19 ( Yin du ), CV-12 ( Zhong wan ), K-21 ( You men )

The accompanying points : ST-44 ( Nei ting ), LI-4 ( He gu ), CV-13 ( Shang wan ), ST-36 ( Zu san li )

SP-4 and PC-6 are a pair of points to treat nausea and vomiting and regulate digestion. Local points are used to reduce pain and regulate the digestive tract. CV-12 is the front Mu alarm point of stomach and Hui meeting point of Fu organs. K-21 and K-19 are used to regulate the digestive tract and also are the local points. LI-7 is the Xi cleft point of large intestine. LI-4 is the Yuan source point of large intestine. SP-4 is needled before PC-6. Strong manipulation is used. ST-34 is the Xi cleft point and it relieve the abdominal pain.

### <48> Gastric atony

Stomach muscles are weak and can not promote the movement of stomach. Medical consultation is essential. The patients have low appetite. Foods remain in stomach for a long time and sometimes there is water sounds when the stomach area is pressed. In severe cases, patients experience dizziness, headache or neurasthenia. The treatment idea is tonifying Qi of spleen and stomach to promote the movement of stomach. The case is usually deficiency case and regular treatment by moxibustion is used.

The main points : GV-20 ( Bai hui ), BL-21 ( Wei shu ), CV-9 ( Shui fen ), CV-14 ( Ju que ), ST-36 ( Zu san li ), CV-4 ( Guan yuan ), CV-12 ( Zhong wan ), CV-10 ( Xia wan )

The accompanying points : SP-3 ( Tai bai ), GV-4 ( Ming men ), BL-20 ( Pi shu ), Liv-13 ( Zhang men ), SP-4 ( Gong sun ), SP-8 ( Di ji ), BL-17 ( Ge shu ), ST-21 ( Liang men )

CV-12 is the front Mu alarm point of stomach. CV-9 eliminates water in stomach, activates the Qi of stomach. Liv-13 is the Hui meeting point of Zang organs and also front Mu alarm point of spleen to tonify organs. ST-36 and BL-21 tonifies Qi of stomach. ST-21 relieve pain and eliminate water and foods from stomach. GV-20 tonifies Qi. SP-8 and BL-17 move blood. Moxibustion is used. Acupuncture can be used for acute case.

### <49> Gastric hyperacidity

Abdominal pain 3 hours after eating. Medical consultation is essential. Usually patients have chest pain, acid belching, pain around CV-14 ( Ju que ). Pain is reduced with eating. Patients have too much appetite. Treatment idea is to reduce the stomach heat and relieve pain.

The main points : Lu-10 ( Yu ji ), ST-44 ( Nei ting ), SP-4 ( Gong sun ), PC-6 ( Nei guan ), ST-36 ( Zu san li ), LI-11 ( Qu chi ), ST-34 ( Liang qiu )

The accompanying points : CV-13 ( Shang wan ), SP-6 ( San yin jiao ), ST-45 ( Li dui ), ST-43 ( Xian gu ), Zhong kui ( Ex ), SP-8 ( Di ji ), CV-12 ( Zhong wan )

Zhong kui is an extra acupoint. The location is at the midpoint of the proximal interphalangeal joint on the dorsal side of the middle finger and it stops vomiting, nausea and hiccups. ST-44 is the Xing spring point of ST channel and that clears the stomach heat. ST-45 is the Jing well point of ST channel that clears the heat. SP-4 and PC-6 are a pair of points to regulate the middle burner problems. Lu-10 is the Ying ( Xing ) spring point that clears the heat of lung and lung is connected with spleen as the Tai yin family group. Spleen is connected with stomach as the same middle burner.

### <50> Gastritis

The main cause is salty foods, stimulating foods, alcohol, excessive eating, too hot or too cold foods. Medical consultation is essential. Mental stress or genetic reason is also the main cause. There are excess syndrome for acute case and deficiency syndrome for chronic case. Symptoms are nausea, vomiting, bloated abdomen, oppressed feeling on stomach, abdominal pain or fever. The treatment idea is regulating middle burner to eliminate the stagnation of heat, coldness or accumulation of phlegm that produce gastritis, tonifying spleen and stomach for deficiency case.

The main points : SP-4 ( Gong sun ), SP-9 ( Yin ling quan ), PC-6 ( Nei guan ), Lu-10 ( Yu ji ), ST-43 ( Xian gu ), ST-36 ( Zu san li ), CV-12 ( Zhong wan ), Liv-3 ( Tai chong ), CV-4 ( Guan yuan )
The accompanying points : BL-20 ( Pi shu ), BL-21 ( Wei shu ), BL-23 ( Shen shu ), LI-4 ( He gu ), CV-13 ( Shang wan ), ST-21 ( Liang men ), CV-10 ( Xia wan ), ST-34 ( Liang qiu )

Lu-10 is the Ying ( Xing ) spring point and treats the spleen and stomach. ST-43 has very good effects on gastritis. SP-4 and PC-6 are a pair of points to regulate the middle burner. ST-36 is lower He sea point and Liv-3 treats the mental stress that causes Gastritis. CV-12 is the front mu alarm point of stomach. BL-21 and BL-20 nourishes spleen and stomach. ST-34 relieves abdominal pain. SP-4 is needled before PC-6. Strong manipulation is used.

### <51> Gastroptosis
This is abnormal downward displacement of the stomach. Medical consultation is essential. The patient can experience chest pain, belching, lower back pain, constipation, vomiting, anorexia, dyspepsia, tenesmus or nausea. The treatment idea is to tonify Qi and direct the Qi upward to hold the stomach.

The main points : Wei shang ( Ex ), Ti wei ( Ex ), Wei luo ( Ex ), ST-36 ( Zu san li ), CV-12 ( Zhong wan ), GV-20 ( Bai hui ), CV-4 ( Guan yuan ), CV-13 ( Shang wan )
The accompanying points : CV-6 ( Qi hai ), GV-4 ( Ming men ), CV-11 ( Jian li ), SP-4 ( Gong sun )

Some special extra points are used. Wei shang is an extra acupoint. The location is at 4 cun lateral from CV-10. Ti wei is an extra acupoint. The location is at 4 cun lateral from CV-12. Wei luo is an extra acupoint. The location is at 4 cun lateral from the point 0.2 cun above CV-9. These three extra acupoints treat the Gastroptosis. The needling direction of Wei shang is to CV-4. ST-36, CV-6 and CV-4 tonify Qi. GV-20 tonifies Qi and direct Qi upwards to hold the stomach. Needling direction is important not to damage liver or other organs. Medium level manipulation is used and moxibustion for chronic case.

### <52> Hemorrhoids

Hemorrhoids are swollen veins in anus or lower rectum, it can develop inside the rectum or around the anus. Medical consultation is essential. The symptoms are swelling on the local, pain, discomfort, itching, red blood in feces. Not all blood in feces are symptoms of hemorrhoids, it can be a symptoms of other diseases like colon cancer or anal cancer. Medical exam is necessary to confirm it. The treatment idea is to activate the circulation of Qi and blood around the anus and rectum. The BL channel is the most related channel for this case because it passes around the anus.

The main points : BL-57 ( Cheng shan ), Liv-3 ( Tai chong ), Er bai ( Ex ), SP-9 ( Yin ling quan ), BL-36 ( Cheng fu ), Lu-6 ( Kong zui ), GV-1 ( Chang qiang ), BL-40 ( Wei zhong ) : bloodletting technique, SP-10 ( Xue hai )

The accompanying points : LI-11 ( Qu chi ), BL-60 ( Kun lun ), LI-4 ( He gu ), ST-37 ( Shang ju xu ), BL-32 ( Ci liao ), SP-8 ( Di ji ), BL-35 ( Hui yang ), BL-30 ( Bai huan shu ), GV-20 ( Bai hui )

Bloodletting technique on BL-40 or the blue vessels around BL-40 is effective. Bloodletting technique on BL-40 is used every week. Er bai is 2 points. they are 4 cun above the wrist line, on both sides of the flexor caparis radialis tendon on the Yin side of the forearms. Er bai is the special extra acupoint for hemorrhoids. The location is at 4 cun above the wrist crease, on both sides of the flexor carpi radialis tendon. BL-30 and GV-1 is the local points to move Qi and blood of the anus and rectum. Lu-6 is the Xi cleft point of Lung to move Qi and blood of large intestine and it stops pains. GV-20 treats hemorrhoids from the top of the head. This follows the principle of correspondence between the top and the bottom. BL-60 is the distant point to regulate the anus and rectum. Eliminating the blood stagnation is dampness is important. Strong manipulation is used for the main points. Moxibustion is more effective on Er bai.

### <53> Hiccup

There are many causes of hiccup. Some chronic diseases like stomach cancer, alcohol addiction or hysteria can cause it. Medical consultation is essential. If the cause is a chronic disease, it is necessary to treat the causing disease at the same time. The prescription here is only for treating the symptom. Hiccup is a symptom of irregularly ascending Qi of stomach. The treatment idea is to regulate Qi of stomach and make the Qi go downwards.

The main points : PC-6 ( Nei guan ), ST-43 ( Xian gu ), CV-22 ( Tian tu ), BL-17 ( Ge shu ), CV-12 ( Zhong wan ), SP-4 ( Gong sun ), ST-36 ( Zu san li )

The accompanying points : LI-11 ( Qu chi ), ST-44 ( Nei ting ), Liv-2 ( Xing jian ), LI-10 ( Shou san li ), LI-4 ( He gu ), ST-37 ( Shang ju xu )

Other method : BL-2 ( Zan zhu ) – electrical acupuncture to maintain the stimulation for about 20-30 min.

SP-4 and PC-6 is a pair of points to regulate the middle burner. CV-22 make the Qi of stomach go downwards. BL17 calms the trembling of diaphragm. CV-12 is the front Mu alarm point of stomach, ST-44 reduces the stomach heat to calm the ascending Qi. Liv-2 reduces the liver heat that was probably influencing the stomach. Needle SP-4 before PC-6. Strong manipulation is used. Strong and continuous stimulation on BL-2 is known to have a function of calming the hiccup.

### <54> Hypochlorhydria

Stomach is not producing enough acid to digest foods. Medical consultation is essential. The possible causes are Weak stomach function, Old age, mal-nutrition, stomach cancer, malign anemia or diabetes etc. The patients experience oppressing feeling on the upper abdomen, nausea, vomiting, loss of appetite or diarrhea and if it gets worse, they can experience headache, loss of desire, nervousness, insomnia or other neural symptoms. Treatment of the causing disease is necessary. The prescription here is only for the symptom. The treatment idea is to activate the function of stomach.

The main points : CV-12 ( Zhong wan ), ST-36 ( Zu san li ), ST-43 ( Xian gu ), BL-50 ( Wei cang ), Liv-14 ( Qi men ), SP-4 ( Gong sun ), PC-6 ( Nei guan ), CV-4 ( Guan yuan ), BL-17 ( Ge shu ), BL-20 ( Pi shu ), BL-21 ( Wei shu )

The accompanying points : GV-4 ( Ming men ), Lu-6 ( Kong zui ), ST-40 ( Feng long ), ST-21 ( Liang men ), SP-6 ( San yin jiao ), GB-34 ( Yang ling quan ), GV-9 ( Zhi yang ), CV-14 ( Ju que ), SP-8 ( Di ji ), GV-20 ( Bai hui )

SP-4 and PC-6 is the pair to activate the spleen and stomach, the middle burner. CV-12, CV-14 are the local points to activate the middle burner. BL-50 activates stomach. GV-9 increases the movement of stomach. BL-17 nourishes blood that may be insufficient for this patient. Lu-6 is the Xi cleft point of lung, and that activates the Qi and blood of lung and large intestine. ST-40 eliminates the possible accumulation of phlegm. Soft manipulation is used.

### <55> Indigestion (1) – diarrhea, fever, vomiting

This case of indigestion is from food intoxication. Medical consultation is essential. The patient experience fever, diarrhea or vomiting. The treatment idea is regulating the middle burner and the lower burner to activate the digestion function, stop diarrhea and pains. ST, LI channel are the main channels.

The main points : Liv-3 ( Tai chong ), ST-36 ( Zu san li ), Lu-5 ( Chi ze ), ST-25 ( Tian shu ), Si feng ( Ex ) : bloodletting technique, LI-11 ( Qu chi ), PC-6 ( Nei guan ), CV-12 ( Zhong wan ), LI-7 ( Wen liu ), Lu-11 ( Shao shang ) : bloodletting technique, SP-4 ( Gong sun ), SP-6 ( San yin jiao )

The accompanying points : CV-6 ( Qi hai ), SP-9 ( Yin ling quan ), ST-44 ( Nei ting ), LI-4 ( He gu ), SP-6 ( San yin jiao ), LI-10 ( Shou san li ), BL-40 ( Wei zhong ), CV-4 ( Guan yuan )

CV-12 is the front Mu alarm point of stomach and it regulates the function of middle burner and stomach. Lu-11 is the Jing well point and can be used for emergency case. LI-7 is the Xi cleft point of large intestine and regulates the spleen and stomach to treat abdominal pain and diarrhea. ST-36 tonifies Qi of spleen and stomach to activate the digestion and eliminate the dampness from food. CV-4 stops diarrhea and regulate the lower burner. ST-25 is the front Mu alarm point of large intestine to stop diarrhea.

### <56> Indigestion (2) – stagnation of food

Eating in hurry, greasy food, excessive eating will be the main causes. Medical consultation is essential. The treatment idea is to relieve the stomach pain, regulate the middle burner, liberate the stagnation of Qi and foods. Jing Well points of hands and feet relieve the emergency situation. Usually bloodletting technique is used for the Jing Well points.

The main points : Lu-11 ( Shao shang ) : bloodletting technique, Liv 3 ( Tai chong ), SP-1 ( Yin bai ), ST-45 ( Li dui ), SP-4 ( Gong sun

), ST-36 ( Zu san li), PC-6 ( Nei guan ), LI-4 ( He gu ), ST-40 ( Feng long )

The accompanying points : LI-11 ( Qu chi ), SP-8 ( Di ji ), ST-37 ( Xia ju xu ), ST-34 ( Liang qiu )

The Jing well points ( SP-1, ST-45, Lu-11 ) relieve the emergency situation of foods stagnation. SP-4 and PC-6 is a pair that regulate the middle burner. ST-34 is the Xi cleft point of ST channel and it relieve the acute pain. ST-36 and ST-37 are the lower He sea points of the stomach and large intestine. ST-40 can eliminate the phlegm and dampness. LI-11 cool the heat that might be from foods stagnation. SP-8 move blood. Strong manipulation is used because it is an acute situation and excess syndrome.

### <57> Intestinal bleeding

Treatment of the causing disease is necessary. Medical consultation is essential. The causing diseases can be intestine cancer, ulcerative colitis, eating spicy foods, ulcer in the digestive tract etc. The prescription here is to treat the symptom. The treatment idea is regulating the lower burner, nourish blood and regulate the blood to stop bleeding.

The main points : GB-36 ( Wai qiu ), LI-2 ( Er jian ), ST-37 ( Shang ju xu ), LI-10 ( Shou san li ), CV-4 ( Guan yuan ), SP-10 ( Xue hai ), ST-44 ( Nei ting ), BL-17 ( Ge shu ), ST-25 ( Tian shu ), SP-8 ( Di ji )

The accompanying points : K-7 ( Fu liu ), BL-25 ( Da chang shu ), GB-34 ( Yang ling quan ), Liv-3 ( Tai chong ), GV-20 ( Bai hui ), ST-36 ( Zu san li ), SP-9 ( Yin ling quan ), BL-27 ( Xiao chang shu )

SP-10 and BL-17 regulate the blood and treat the blood problem. SP-9 eliminates dampness and tonifies spleen. ST-25 is the front Mu alarm point of large intestine. ST-37 is the lower He sea point of large intestine. GV-20 holds the blood not to bleed.

### <58> Intestinal obstruction, ileus

This is an emergency and risk situation. Medical consultation is essential. It is necessary to send the patient to the emergency hospital. The patient can experience severe abdominal pain, difficulty in eliminating gas, palpable mass in the lower abdomen and constipation. The treatment idea is to regulate the movement of intestine to relieve its obstruction. The emergency points are used.

The main points : ST-25 ( Tian shu ), SP-14 ( Fu jie ), SP-15 ( Da heng ), CV-4 ( Guan yuan ), LI-7 ( Wen liu ), ST-37 ( Shang ju xu ), ST-39 ( Xia ju xu ), ST-36 ( Zu san li ), PC-6 ( Nei guan )

The accompanying points : BL-23 ( Shen shu ), BL-27 ( Xiao chang shu ), LI-11 ( Qu chi ), CV-6 ( Qi hai ), BL-25 ( Da chang shu ), CV-12 ( Zhong wan )

Xi cleft points directly influence the Qi and blood of the organ and are used for acute situations. LI-7 is the Xi cleft point of large intestine. The local points around lower abdomen are used to regulate the intestine. ST-37 is the lower He sea point of large intestine. CV-4 and CV-6 regulate the movement of intestine. BL-23 and BL-27 generate Qi and move Qi in the lower burner. Strong manipulation is used.

### <59> Intestinal stenosis, enterostenosis

This is a narrowing of the passage within the small or large intestine. Medical consultation is essential. The patients experience bloated abdomen, abdominal pains or diarrhea. The treatment idea is to activating the functions of intestine to widen its passage.

The main points : CV-12 ( Zhong wan ), TB-6 ( Zhi gou ), ST-25 ( Tian shu ), ST-37 ( Shang ju xu ), LI-7 ( Wen liu ), CV-4 ( Guan yuan ), ST-36 ( Zu san li), BL-25 ( Da chang shu ), SP-14 ( Fu jie, Left side )

The accompanying points : LI-4 ( He gu ), LI-10 ( Shou san li ), LI-11 ( Qu chi ), Liv-3 ( Tai chong ), ST-39 ( Xia ju xu ), Ht-7 ( Shen men ), GB-28 ( Wei dao, Left side ), ST-43 ( Xian gu )

CV-12 is the front Mu alarm point of stomach. ST-25 is the front Mu alarm point of large intestine. ST-37 and ST-39 are the lower He sea point of the large intestine and small intestine. LI-4 and Liv-3 are used to relieve the muscle stress and pain. CV-4 and other points around lower abdomen activate the movement of intestine. Needles and moxibustion can be used together.

**<60> Intestinal tuberculosis**
Intestine has the tuberculosis. Medical consultation is essential. The patients experience diarrhea in the early morning, constipation, abdominal pain, fatigue, loss of appetite or bloated abdomen. The treatment idea is to tonify the Qi and Yang of kidneys and spleen to activate the intestine and spleen.

The main points : ST-36 ( Zu san li ), CV-8 ( Shen que, Do not needle ) : moxibustion, ST-25 ( Tian shu ), ST-44 ( Nei ting ), K-16 ( Huang shu ), CV-4 ( Guan yuan ), K-6 ( Zhao hai ), SP-4 ( Gong sun ), BL-25 ( Da chang shu ), SP-6 ( San yin jiao )
The accompanying points : GV-20 ( Bai hui ), K-7 ( Fu liu ), BL-60 ( Kun lun ), CV-6 ( Qi hai ), BL-33 ( Zhong liao ), ST-34 ( Liang qiu )

CV-4, CV-6, ST-25, CV-8 and K-16 regulate and activate the intestine. CV-4 and CV-6 tonifies the Qi of Kidneys and regulate the intestine. ST-34 relieves the abdominal pains. GV-20 tonifies Qi and hold the Qi not to go downwards and stops diarrhea. K-7 tonifies kidneys. SP-6 nourishes Yin and Qi of spleen, liver and kidneys. Moxibustion is used on abdomen.

**<61> Loss of appetite**
This is a common symptom. Medical consultation is essential. There can be many causing diseases of digestive tract or it can happen simply because of emotional stress or neurosis. The treatment idea is activating digestive tract and relieve mental and emotional stress.

The main points : ST-25 ( Tian shu ), SP-4 ( Gong sun ), SP-6 ( San yin jiao ), CV-4 ( Guan yuan ), LI-11 ( Qu chi ), CV-12 ( Zhong wan ), ST-21 ( Liang men ), PC-6 ( Nei guan ), ST-36 ( Zu san li ), GV-20 ( Bai hui )

The accompanying points : Ht-7 ( Shen men ), SP-8 ( Di ji ), BL-18 ( Gan shu ), BL-50 ( Wei cang ), BL-20 ( Pi shu ), BL-21 ( Wei shu ), LI-10 ( Shou san li ), Liv-3 ( Tai chong ), LI-4 ( He gu )

PC-6 and SP-4 is a good pair of points that treats the problem of middle burner and promotes digestion as well. ST-36 promotes digestion and tonifies spleen and stomach to have more appetite. ST-21 eliminates the foods in the stomach rapidly. Liv-3 and LI-4 relieve mental stress and also promote digestion. CV-4 warms the spleen and stomach to activate them. Ht-7 is for mental or emotional causes. Medium level manipulation is used.

### <62> Nausea and vomiting (1)

These symptoms are related with diseases of stomach or intestine but it also can happen with neurosis, emotional problems, parasite or pregnancy etc. Medical consultation is essential. Most of all, treating the causing disease is necessary. In TCM, nausea and vomiting is phenomenon of irregularly ascending stomach Qi. The treatment idea is to regulate the stomach Qi and calm the irregularly ascending stomach Qi. There are heat or coldness syndrome, excess or deficiency syndrome.

The main points : Lu-10 ( Yu ji ), SP-4 ( Gong sun ), PC-6 ( Nei guan ), CV-12 ( Zhong wan ), ST-44 ( Nei ting ), ST-36 ( Zu san li ), SP-9 ( Yin ling quan ), CV-22 ( Tian tu )

The accompanying points : TB-2 ( Ye men ), CV-13 ( Shang wan ), SP-6 ( San yin jiao ), BL-21 ( Wei shu ), LI-4 ( He gu ), Ht-7 ( Shen men ), GV-20 ( Bai hui ), CV-4 ( Guan yuan )

ST-36, SP-4 and PC-6 calm the ascending stomach Qi. CV-22 also has the strong function to calm the ascending stomach Qi. Lu-10 and ST-44 clears the lung and stomach heat. CV-4 tonifies kidneys Yang to warm the stomach in case the stomach is cold. Ht-7 calm the mind for emotional cause. GV-20 calms the mind and also regulate the movement of Qi. TB-2 clears the heat from TB and regulate the function of triple burner.

### <63> Nausea and Vomiting (2)

These symptoms are related with diseases of stomach or intestine but it also can happen with neurosis, emotional problems, parasite or pregnancy etc. Medical consultation is essential. Most of all, treating the causing disease is necessary. In TCM, nausea and vomiting is phenomenon of irregularly ascending stomach Qi. The treatment idea is to regulate the stomach Qi and calm the irregularly ascending stomach Qi. There are heat or coldness syndrome, excess or deficiency syndrome.

The main points : ST-36 ( Zu san li ), ST-44 ( Nei ting ), PC-6 ( Nei guan ), CV-13 ( Shang wan ), CV-12 ( Zhong wan ), CV-17 ( Shan zhong )
The accompanying points : Ht-7 ( Shen men ), Liv-2 ( Xing jian ), LI-4 ( He gu ), BL-21 ( Wei shu ), TB-5 ( Wai guan )
If pregnancy is the cause of disease : PC-6 ( Nei guan ).

PC-6 makes the movement of Qi go downwards. CV-12, CV-13 regulate the middle burner. ST-44 clears the stomach heat that may be the cause of the symptoms. TB-5 opens the TB channel to help the Qi flow up and down. BL-21 and ST-36 regulate stomach. In case of mental stress, relieving stagnation of liver Qi is necessary. Medium level manipulation is used.

### <64> Prolapse of anus

The main cause of this problem is deficiency of Qi, that makes Qi ascension difficult. Medical consultation is essential. The treatment idea is to tonify Qi, elevate the movement of Qi upwards.

The main points : ST-37 ( Shang ju xu ), CV-6 ( Qi hai ), CV-4 ( Guan yuan ), GV-20 ( Bai hui ), BL-57 ( Cheng shan ), GV-12 ( Shen zhu ), GV-1 ( Chang qiang )

The accompanying points : LI-4 ( He gu ), ST-25 ( Tian shu ), ST-36 ( Zu san li ), BL-30 ( Bai huan shu ), BL-33 ( Zhong liao ), LI-11 ( Qu chi ), LI-7 ( Wen liu )

GV-1 is the special point for prolapse of anus. CV-6 and GV-20 tonifies Qi. GV-20 holds the Qi not to fall downwards. GV-12 tonifies Qi. If too many needles are used, the patient will lose Qi. It is better use proper number of needles to tonify Qi. Strong manipulation is used for the points near anus and soft manipulation is used for distant points to tonify Qi. Moxibustion can be used for the distant points.

### <65> Stomach ache – acute case

There are many causes but the most common causes are gastritis, mental stress or stimulating foods intake. Medical consultation is essential. The symptoms are local pain, bloated abdomen, fever or nausea and vomiting. The treatment idea of this prescription is to regulate middle burner and stop pains.

The main points : ST-21 ( Liang men ), ST-45 ( Li Dui ), ST-36 ( Zu san li ), SP-4 ( Gong sun ), PC-6 ( Nei guan ), ST-34 ( Liang qiu ), CV-12 ( Zhong wan, indirect soft warm moxibustion )

The accompanying points : LI-4 ( He gu ), SP-8 ( Di ji ), CV-15 ( Jiu wei ), Liv-3 ( Tai chong ), GV-20 ( Bai hui )

ST-34 is the Xi cleft point of ST channel that moves Qi and blood of the channel and stops stomach pains. ST-45 is the Jing well point of ST channel and it is used for emergency cases. SP-4 and PC-6 are a pair to regulate the middle burner. SP-4 has to be needled before PC-6. SP-8 eliminate the blood stasis. Warm and soft moxibustion around CV-12 can be applied to relieve pain. GV-20, LI-4 and Liv-3 relieve mental stress and muscle tension. Strong manipulation for ST-34 is used. Bloodletting technique is used for ST-45.

### <66> Stomach cancer

A medical consultation with an oncology specialist in a hospital is essential for all cancer cases. Acupuncture is for relieving pain and improving symptoms only. Avoid the points on the tumor or too near the tumor. In China, a combination of TCM herbal medicine and Western medical treatment is commonly used for oncology cases. The management idea of this prescription is to regulate middle burner to relieve pain and symptoms, tonify Qi and move Qi and blood. Be careful not to needle the tumor itself. If the development of cancer or metastasis is severe, acupuncture is not used. You can refer to the section that discusses cancer cases, which is located in the final part of this book.

The main points : Liv-3 ( Tai chong ), CV-4 ( Guan yuan ), CV-12 ( Zhong wan ) : do not needle and use moxibustion, ST-36 ( Zu san li ), BL-50 ( Wei cang ), ST-19 ( Bu rong ) : do not needle and use moxibustion, CV-14 ( Ju que ) : do not needle and use moxibustion, SP-4 ( Gong sun ), PC-6 ( Nei guan ), CV-6 ( Qi hai )

The accompanying points : BL-17 ( Ge shu ), LI-4 ( He gu ), CV-13 ( Shang wan ) : do not needle, use moxibustion, CV-10 ( Xia wan ) : do not needle, use moxibustion, ST-40 ( Feng long ), Liv-13 ( Zhang men ), BL-21 ( Wei shu ), GV-20 ( Bai hui )

CV-12 is the front Mu alarm point of stomach, BL-21 is the back shu point of stomach. LI-4 and Liv-3 relieve mental stress and pain. BL-17 nourishes blood. PC-6 and SP-4 regulate the middle burner. Medium level manipulation is used. Be careful not to needle the tumor itself ( be careful with CV-12 ). The moxibustion is used for the deficiency of Yang and Qi.

### <67> Stomach spasm, gastrospasm

The sudden and severe pain on stomach is the main symptom. Medical consultation is essential. There are many causes but the most common ones are mental and emotional shock or stimulating foods. The treatment idea is to use Xi cleft point to relieve acute pain, regulate the middle burner and move Qi and blood to relieve tension and spasm.

The main points : PC-6 ( Nei guan ), GB-31 ( Feng shi ), BL-17 ( Ge shu ), SP-8 ( Di ji ), ST-36 ( Zu san li ), SP-4 ( Gong sun ), Liv-3 ( Tai chong ), ST-34 ( Liang qiu )

The accompanying points : GB-34 ( Yang ling quan ), BL-18 ( Gan shu ), ST-44 ( Nei ting ), BL-21 ( Wei shu ), BL-19 ( Dan shu ), BL-20 ( Pi shu ), GV-20 ( Bai hui )

ST-34 is the Xi cleft point of stomach and it stops pain. Liv-3 and BL-17 move blood to relieve the tension and calm the wind. SP-4 and PC-6 are a pair to regulate the middle burner. The accompanying points are back shu points of Liv, GB, SP and ST. They harmonize the organs to treat the spasm. Strong manipulation is used. Because the patient is in emergency situation and can move body for pain, the needles have to be removed soon after the manipulation.

### <68> Stomach ulcer

The symptoms are stomach pain, vomiting blood or gastric hyperacidity. Medical consultation is essential. The treatment idea is to regulate the middle burner, eliminate the inflammation and ulcer at the local area.

The main points : BL-21 ( Wei shu ), ST-36 ( Zu san li ), SP-4 ( Gong sun ), PC-6 ( Nei guan ), ST-44 ( Nei ting ), CV-12 ( Zhong wan, indirect soft and warm moxibustion ), Liv-3 ( Tai chong ), ST-21 ( Liang men )

The accompanying points : GV-20 ( Bai hui ), SP-8 ( Di ji ), CV-13 ( Shang wan ), CV-10 ( Xia wan ), CV-14 ( Ju que ), BL-20 ( Pi shu )

The local points around the upper abdomen are selected to calm the stomach and relieve pain. SP-4 and PC-6 regulate the middle burner to relieve the pain. SP-8 moves blood, GB-34 relieve the muscle and tendon tension. ST-44 cool the stomach heat. Long term moxibustion can be used for the points.

# | 11 |

# Ear, nose and throat ( ENT )

**<69> Auditory vertigo, Meniere syndrome**
The cause is a disorder of the inner ear. The main symptoms are dizziness, hearing loss, tinnitus and feeling fullness of the ear. Medical consultation is essential. The treatment idea is to eliminate the internal wind, calm the mind, transform the phlegm ( those may be the direct cause ), nourish kidneys to prevent the wind, open orifice ( ears ) and regulate the Qi and blood around the ear.

The main points : BL-23 ( Shen shu ), K-7 ( Fu liu ), TB-3 ( Zhong zhu ), CV-9 ( Shui fen ), TB-2 ( Ye men ), GB-41 ( Zu lin qi ), SI-19 ( Ting gong ), GB-20 ( Feng chi ), TB-17 ( Yi feng ), PC-6 ( Nei guan ), SP-9 ( Yin ling quan ), Tai yang ( Ex )
The accompanying points : GB-2 ( Ting hui ), An mian ( Ex ), K-3 ( Tai xi ), CV-12 ( Zhong wan ), ST-40 ( Feng long ), GV-26 ( Shui gou ), BL-60 ( Kun lun ), BL-7 ( Tong tian ), Liv-2 ( Xing jian ) or Liv-3 ( Tai chong ), GV-20 ( Bai hui )

The Liv and GB channel points eliminate the internal wind. Especially GB-20 has the strong function to pacify the internal wind. PC-6 transforms phlegm and opens orifice. TB-2 and TB-3 are the distant points to activate ears. Tai yang is at the lateral sides of the head and it activates the local movement of Qi and blood with BL-7. K-7 and K-3 nourish kidneys to calm the wind. An mian is the extra acupoint and the location is at the middle point between the TB-17 and GB-20, that calms the mind and wind. BL-60 lowers the floating Yang and pacifies the internal wind. ST-40 and CV-12 transforms phlegm. GV-26 opens the orifice. Strong manipulation is used for the local area of ear and head.

### <70> Deaf-mutism, surdimutism

This is difficulty in hearing and speaking. Usually if the deafness happens in the early age, the patients have a difficulty in learning how to speak and will have mutism. Medical consultation is essential. There are many causes like hereditary reason and diseases. The treatment idea is to activate the movement of Qi and blood of ears, nourish kidneys, pacify the internal wind, open orifice to clear the head and increase the perception.

The main points : K-3 ( Tai xi ), GV-26 ( Shui gou ), TB-21 ( Er men ), Liv-3 ( Tai chong ), SI-19 ( Ting gong ), GB-20 ( Feng chi ), TB-17 ( Yi feng ), K-7 ( Fu liu ), SI-3 ( Hou xi ), GB-2 ( Ting hui ), GV-15 ( Ya men ), TB-3 ( Zhong zhu )

The accompanying points : BL-23 ( Shen shu ), TB-5 ( Wai guan ), GV-20 ( Bai hui ), GB-41 ( Zu lin qi ), LI-4 ( He gu ), PC-6 ( Nei guan ), BL-10 ( Tian zhu )

GB-20, TB-17 pacify the internal wind. K-7, K-3 and SI-3 nourish the kidneys and ear. SI-19, GB-2, TB-21 are the local points around the ears to activate the movement of Qi and blood around the ears. GV-15 influences the brain and activates the speaking function. PC-6 and GV-26 open orifices to clear the head and ears. TB-5 regulates the ears. Strong manipulation is used for the local points near ears and orifices opening points. Soft manipulation is used for points that tonify kidneys

### <71> Deafness (1) – sequelae of a disease.

This is about difficulty in hearing. The common causes are inflammation at internal ears, auditory nerves or ageing of auditory nerves etc. Medical consultation is essential. The treatment idea is to eliminate the pathogens at the ear and treat the inflammation, regulate the Qi and blood of the ear, pacify the internal wind and nourish kidneys to prevent and treat the deafness. The local and distant points are used.

The main points : GB-31 ( Feng shi ), SI-19 ( Ting gong ), TB-21 ( Er men ), K-7 ( Fu liu ), BL-23 ( Shen shu ), GB-41 ( Zu lin qi ), GB-2 ( Ting hui ), TB-17 ( Yi feng ), GB-20 ( Feng chi ), TB-3 ( Zhong zhu ), SI-3 ( Hou xi ), TB-5 ( Wai guan )

The accompanying points : K-3 ( Tai xi ), Liv-3 ( Tai chong ), GB-43 ( Xia xi ), GB-34 ( Yang ling quan ), LI-4 ( He gu )

GB-41 and TB-5 are a pair of points to treat and regulate the lateral sides of the head including ears. TB-17 and GB-20 pacify the internal wind and clears the head. TB-3, K-7, BL-23 nourish the kidneys and activate the ear. GB-43 clears the heat of GB channel. LI-4 is for the problem of head. SI-3 and K-3 nourish and activate kidneys and ears. Medium level manipulation is used.

### <72> Deafness (2) – sequelae of a disease

This is about difficulty in hearing. The common causes are inflammation at internal ears, auditory nerves or ageing of auditory nerves etc. Medical consultation is essential. The treatment idea is to eliminate the pathogens at the ear and treat the inflammation, regulate the Qi and blood of the ear, pacify the internal wind and nourish kidneys to prevent and treat the deafness. The local and distant points are used.

The main points : TB-5 ( Wai guan ), K-3 ( Tai xi ), BL-23 ( Shen shu ), TB-21 ( Er men ), GB-2 ( Ting hui ), TB-2 ( Ye men ), SI-19 (

Ting gong ), TB-17 ( Yi feng ), GB-44 ( Zu qiao yin ), GB-20 ( Feng chi )

The accompanying points : GB-21 ( Jian jing ), Liv-2 ( Xing jian ), GB-41 ( Zu lin qi ), TB-3 ( Zhong zhu ), K-7 ( Fu liu ), Ht-3 ( Shao hai ),

TB-17, SI-19, TB-21 and GB-2 eliminate the pathogen around the ears. GB-41 and TB-5 are a pair for ears. BL-23 nourishes the kidneys. TB-2 and TB-3 activate the Qi and blood around the ears. K-7 nourishes kidneys, Ht-3 clears the heat of heart. GB-21 regulates the Qi. Medium level or soft manipulation is used.

<73> **Ear pain**

This symptom can happen with various diseases of ears, suppurative inflammation or otitis media. Medical consultation is essential. It is necessary to treat the causing diseases as well. The treatment idea is to clear the heat in the TB channels and regulate the Qi and blood of ear.

The main points : TB-17 ( Yi feng ), K-7 ( Fu liu ), SI-19 ( Ting gong ), GB-3 ( Shang guan ), GB-20 ( Feng chi ), TB-2 ( Ye men ), PC-4 ( Xi men ), K-3 ( Tai xi ), TB-21 ( Er men )

The accompanying points : TB-9 ( Si du ), Liv-2 ( Xing jian ), TB-16 ( Tian you ), SI-3 ( Hou xi ), GB-43 ( Xia xi ), SI-17 ( Tian rong ), BL-10 ( Tian zhu ), GB-2 ( Ting hui ),

The local points are used to regulate the local Qi and blood. TB-2 clears the heat of TB channel that passes the ears. TB-9 is the distant point for ears. GB-43 clears the heat of GB channel to eliminate the inflammation of ears. GB-20 eliminate the wind that may be the cause of pain. Strong manipulation is used for excess syndrome.

<74> **Epistaxis**

This is about bleeding from nose. There are many different causes. Medical consultation is essential. The treatment of the causing diseases is necessary to cure epistaxis completely. The most common cause is the ascending excess heat and the treatment idea is to direct the heat downwards, clear the head and regulate the Qi and blood that flows in the head and nose. This prescription is to treat the symptom only.

The main points : GV-23 ( Shang xing ), ST-37 ( Shang ju xu ), SP-10 ( Xue hai ), GV-16 ( Feng fu ), BL-17 ( Ge shu ), Lu-6 ( Kong zui ), GB-22 ( Xin hui ), Yin tang ( Ex ), LI-4 ( He gu )

The accompanying points : Liv-2 ( Xing jian ), TB-8 ( San yang luo ), BL-13 ( Fei shu ), BL-10 ( Tian zhu ), GV-12 ( Shen zhu ), GV-14 ( Da zhui ), LI-11 ( Qu chi )

Yin tang is the extra acupoint and the location is at the middle point between the two eyebrows. Yin tang and GV-23 are used together to regulate the nose. Lu-6 is the Xi cleft point of lung to stop bleeding. BL-17 is the Hui meeting point of blood to regulate the blood and stop epistaxis. SP-10 regulate the blood. LI-11 clears the Yang ming heat. GV-14 clears the heat. Strong manipulation is used for excess syndrome.

### <75> Esophageal stenosis

The esophageal passage becomes narrow and the patients experience difficulty of swallowing foods and discomfort feeling on the throat. Medical consultation is essential. There is a possibility of tumor and it is necessary to check if it is benign or malignant in the medical exam. One of the common cause is emotional stress. The treatment of neurosis ( emotional stress ) is necessary in the separate session of acupuncture. This prescription is to widen the esophagus and regulate the throat to treat difficult swallowing, nausea and vomiting.

The main points : SP-4 ( Gong sun ), CV-12 ( Zhong wan ), ST-36 ( Zu san li ), LI-4 ( He gu ), ST-40 ( Feng long ), GV-20 ( Bai hui ), PC-6 ( Nei guan ), CV-22 ( Tian tu ), CV-17 ( Shan zhong ), K-6 ( Zhao hai ), Ht-7 ( Shen men )

The accompanying points : GV-12 ( Shen zhu ), CV-14 ( Ju que ), Lu-7 ( Lie que ), Liv-3 ( Tai chong ), LI-11 ( Qu chi ), BL-18 ( Gan shu ), BL-17 ( Ge shu ),

CV-22 directs the Qi downwards. CV-17 eliminates the accumulation of phlegm in chest. PC-6 and SP-4 regulate the digestion. Lu-7 and K-6 regulate the throat. CV-12 and ST-40 activate digestion and transform phlegm. BL-18, Liv-3 and LI-4 eliminate the liver Qi stagnation to relieve emotional stress. BL-17 activates diaphragm for swallowing. The medium level manipulation is used.

### <76> Esophagus spasms

Esophagus becomes contracted and spasms happen. The patients experience sudden, severe, and squeezing pains on chest or burning sensation on chest. Medical consultation is essential. The pain lasts for minutes to hours. The symptom that patients experience is similar to angina pectoris. Medical exam is necessary to check if it is heart problem or esophagus problem. It influences eating. The medical cause is not much known. In TCM the main cause is irregular movement of Qi in chest. The treatment idea is to regulate the Qi in esophagus and stomach.

The main points : ST-36 ( Zu san li ), Ht-7 ( Shen men ), GB-34 ( Yang ling quan ), CV-22 ( Tian tu ), CV-12 ( Zhong wan ), PC-6 ( Nei guan ), SP-4 ( Gong sun ), ST-40 ( Feng long ),

The accompanying points : ST-34 ( Liang qiu ), LI-11 ( Qu chi ), Liv-3 ( Tai chong ), CV-17 ( Shan zhong ), CV-15 ( Jiu wei ), SP-6 ( San yin jiao ),

CV-22 and ST-36 direct the Qi downwards. PC-6 and SP-4 regulate the Qi in chest. CV-12 and CV-15 are the local points. Liv-3 and GB-34 relieve the muscle tension on esophagus. ST-34 is the Xi cleft point of stomach for emergency situation. SP-6 regulates the throat. The strong manipulation is used.

### <77> Goiter

This is an irregular growth of thyroid glands. It may be an overall enlargement or irregular cell growth. It is necessary to check if the enlarged part is benign or malignant. Medical consultation is essential. One of the most common causes is a lack of iodine in diet. Especially the places far from sea easily become in lack of iodine in foods. Taking iodine is the treatment for that case. Other cases are related with emotional stress, thyroid gland problem and other endocrine problems etc. In TCM, goiter is combinational accumulation of Qi and phlegm. The treatment is to regulate the Qi and transform the phlegm in the local area.

The main points : ST-40 ( Feng long ), CV-12 ( Zhong wan ), Lu-7 ( Lie que ), TB-3 ( Zhong zhu ), LI-4 ( He gu ), CV-22 ( Tian tu ), Qi ying ( Ex ), Liv-3 ( Tai chong )

The accompanying points : LI-11 ( Qu chi ), ST-9 ( Ren ying ), Jia ji ( Ex, C3~C5 ), K-6 ( Zhao hai ), GB-20 ( Feng chi ), PC-4 ( Nei guan ),

Qi ying is the extra acupoint for goiter. The location is above clavicle near ST-10. Qi ying is the local point. CV-22 directs the Qi downwards and transforms phlegm. ST-40 transforms phlegm and regulates the Qi movements. Jia ji is the extra acupoints located 0.5 ~ 1cun lateral to the depressions below the spinous processes of the vertebrae. In this prescription the Jia ji that corresponds to C3~C7 are used. Liv-3 and LI-4 improve emotional stress. The accompanying points relieve stress, transform phlegm, regulate the Qi and eliminate the wind. The needles are removed after the manipulation.

### <78> Olfactory disorder, dysosmia

This is a change in the ability to smell. Parosmia is that the smell of a familiar object has changed. Medical consultation is essential. Phantosmia is to smell something that doesn't exist. There are many causes like nasal polyps, hay fever, parkin's disease, smoking, sinusitis, chemotherapy, virus ( infection ) or brain injury etc. The treatment idea is to open orifices, regulate the Qi and blood of nose and open the LI, GV channels to activate the perception.

The main points : Bi tong ( Ex, Shang ying xiang ), PC-6 ( Nei guan ), LI-20 ( Ying xiang ), GV-23 ( Shang xing ), GV-26 ( Shui gou ), SP-9 ( Yin ling quan ), LI-4 ( He gu ), LI-11 ( Qu chi ), LI-19 ( Kou he liao ), BL-67 ( Zhi yin ), LI-1 ( Shang yang )

The accompanying points : ST-40 ( Feng long ), ST-36 ( Zu san li ), BL-10 ( Tian zhu ), Lu-11 ( Shao shang ), GB-20 ( Feng chi ), Yin tang ( Ex ),

Bi tong is at the junction of the maxilla and the nasal cavity, near the upper end of the nasolabial groove. LI-20, Bi tong ( Ex ) and LI-19 are near nose and increase the olfactory perception. LI-11 is the distant point of nose. Yin tang is at the middle point between the two eyebrows. The combination of Yin tang and GV-23 is used to clear the inflammation and open the channel of nose. GV-26 activates the brain and opens orifice. BL-67 is the distant point to regulate the Qi and blood of nose.

### <79> Otitis media – OME ( Otitis media with effusion )

This type of otitis media does not have the typical symptoms except occasional feeling of fullness in the ear. Medical consultation is essential. There is non-infectious fluid in the middle ear after the period of acute otitis media. The treatment idea is to eliminate the phlegm and inflammation of the middle ear.

The main points : GB-20 ( Feng chi ), Liv-2 ( Xing jian ), TB-16 ( Tian you ), TB-17 ( Yi feng ), LI-11 ( Qu chi ), GB-41 ( Zu lin qi ), GB-43 ( Xia xi ), K-2 ( Ran gu ), ST-40 ( Feng long )

The accompanying points : LI-4 ( He gu ), TB-2 ( Ye men ), SI-4 ( Wan gu ), GB-34 ( Yang ling quan ), SI-19 ( Ting gong ), BL-23 ( Shen shu ), TB-5 ( Wai guan ), TB-20 ( Jiao sun )

The local points of ear are used to eliminate the inflammation and to activate the movement of Qi and blood. GB-20 eliminates the wind. GB-43 is the distant point to clear the heat in the GB channel that passes the ear. LI-4 and LI-11 clear the heat. K-2 is the Xing spring point to clear the heat from K channel. ST-40 transforms phlegm and eliminates pus. BL-23 tonifies kidneys and Qi. Strong manipulation is used for acute or excess syndrome. Medium level manipulation is used for chronic situation.

### <80> Otitis media – CSOM ( Chronic suppurative otitis media )

The tympanic membrane is perforated and there is persistent purulent discharge through a perforated tympanic membrane for more than 2 weeks. Medical consultation is essential. At the acute period, usually there had fever but after the purulent discharge is drained, the fever disappears and becomes a chronic case. It is not easily cured. The treatment idea is to activate the Qi and blood around the ear to eliminate the discharge and chronic inflammation. In case there is persistent discharge from the middle ear but there is no fever, it is usually diagnosed as deficiency syndrome.

The main points : K-7 ( Fu liu ), TB-17 ( Yi feng ), LI-11 ( Qu chi ), SI-17 ( Tian rong ), TB-22 ( He liao ), TB-21 ( Er men ), GB-2 ( Ting hui ), TB-5 ( Wai guan ), K-3 ( Tai xi ), SP-9 ( Yin ling quan ), ST-40 ( Feng long )

The accompanying points : ST-36 ( Zu san li ), TB-20 ( Jiao sun ), BL-23 ( Shen shu ), GB-20 ( Feng chi ), TB-2 ( Ye men ), GB-44 ( Zu qiao yin ), SI-19 ( Ting gong ), SI-4 ( Wan gu ), TB-3 ( Zhong zhu ), LI-4 ( He gu ),

The local and distant points in SI, TB and GB channels are used to eliminate the inflammation in the ear. ST-40 transforms phlegm to eliminate discharge. SP-9 dries the dampness and eliminates discharge. K-3 tonifies kidneys Qi to eliminate the discharge and increase the Qi. ST-36 tonifies Qi to recover early. GB-20 eliminates the wind. TB-2 and TB-3 eliminates the inflammation in the ear. In case there is fever, LI-4 and LI-11 can be added. If there is acute fever, strong manipulation is used. If it is chronic and deficiency syndrome, medium level manipulation or indirect moxibustion around the ear can be used.

### <81> Pharyngitis, sore throat

This is the inflammation on throat. It usually happens with common cold, influenza or external infection. Medical consultation is essential. It is usually accompanied by the inflammation of nose. The treatment idea is to clear the heat, relieve the inflammation and detoxify.

The main points : Lu-9 ( Tai yuan ), LI-1 ( Shang yang ), Lu-10 ( Yu ji ), K-6 ( Zhao hai ), Lu-11 ( Shao shang ), LI-11 ( Qu chi ), Lu-5 ( Chi ze ), CV-22 ( Tian tu )
The accompanying points :, ST-44 ( Nei ting ), SP-6 ( San yin jiao ), K-7 ( Fu liu ), Lu-7 ( Lie que ), K-6 ( Zhao hai ), LI-4 ( He gu )

Lu-10 is the Xing spring point to clear the heat from Lung. The pair of Lu-7 and K-6 treats the sore throat. The bloodletting technique is used for LI-1 and Lu-11 to clear the heat from the throat. LI-4 and LI-11 is for the general body fever and infection. SP-6 nourishes the dry throat. Lu-5 eliminates the lung heat. ST-44 clears the body heat.

### <82> Rhinitis by common cold

This is the inflammation on nose with common cold. Medical consultation is essential. The symptoms are headache, insomnia, fever, sensation of coldness, nose blockage, sneeze, fatigue, low appetite, clean phlegm etc. The treatment idea is to clear the fever, eliminate the cold, open the nose and transform the phlegm. In case it becomes chronic case, there are only symptoms of rhinitis without fever and usually the deficiency syndrome is diagnosed. This prescription is for excess syndrome and you can add points to tonify Qi for deficiency and chronic case.

The main points : Lu-7 ( Lie que ), ST-40 ( Feng long ), Yin tang ( Ex ), GV-23 ( Shang xing ), LI-4 ( He gu ), K-6 ( Zhao hai ), LI-11 ( Qu chi ), LI-20 ( Ying xiang ), ST-36 ( Zu san li )

The accompanying points : Liv-2 ( Xing jian ), LI-19 ( Kou he liao ), GB-31 ( Feng shi ), Lu-10 ( Yu ji ), BL-23 ( Shen shu ), BL-67 ( Zhi yin ), Bi tong ( Ex, Shang ying xiang ), CV-12 ( Zhong wan )

Lu-10 is to clear the heat from lung, Lu-7 to eliminate the inflammation from lung. GV-23 and Yin tang is for regulate the nose and opens the orifice. LI-20 open the nose. CV-12 regulates the nose and eliminate the phlegm. ST-40 transforms phlegm. ST-36 directs the Qi downwards. BL-67 causes to Qi descend. Yin tang is at the middle point between the eyebrows. Bi tong is at the junction of the maxilla and the nasal cavity, near the upper end of the nasolabial groove. Strong manipulation is used. Bloodletting technique is used for BL-67.

### <83> Runny nose

There are many causes for runny nose. Medical consultation is essential. First of all, it is necessary to treat the causing diseases. This prescription is for symptoms only. The treatment idea is to activate the functions of lung to open the nose and transform the phlegm.

The main points : LI-20 ( Ying xiang ), Lu-7 ( Lie que ), Lu-6 ( Kong zui ), GB-20 ( Feng chi ), Bi tong ( Ex, Shang ying xiang ), GV-23 ( Shang xing ), ST-36 ( Zu san li ), Yin tang ( Ex ), ST-40 ( Feng long ), SP-9 ( Yin ling quan ), BL-63 ( Jin men )

The accompanying points : LI-11 ( Qu chi ), GB-31 ( Feng shi ), Lu-5 ( Chi ze ), GB-15 ( Tou lin qi ), K-6 ( Zhao hai ), Bi zhu ( Ex ), Liv-2 ( Xing jian ), BL-10 ( Tian zhu ), Bi liu ( Ex ), LI-4 ( He gu )

Yin tang is at the middle point between the two eyebrows. Bi tong is at the junction of the maxilla and the nasal cavity, near the upper end of the nasolabial groove and it opens the nose with LI-20. ST-40 and SP-9 eliminate the dampness and phlegm. BL-63 pacifies the wind. Lu-5 reduces the Lu channel. Bi liu and Bi zhu are just under the nose. They open the orifice of nose. Lu-5 reduces the excess syndrome of lung. Strong manipulation is used.

### <84> Sinusitis

There are acute or chronic cases. Medical consultation is essential. The symptoms are persistent discharge from the tissue lining sinuses, nose blockage or headache etc. This is an inflammation of the tissue lining sinuses. The treatment idea is to eliminate the brain heat that is causing the inflammation of sinuses, open the orifice of nose, regulate the Qi and blood around the sinuses and nose and transform the phlegm. There are cold or heat syndromes. Following the syndromes you can add the points.

The main points : K-6 ( Zhao hai ), Lu-7 ( Lie que ), Liv-2 ( Xing jian ), GV-23 ( Shang xing ), BL-7 ( Tong tian ), LI-11 ( Qu chi ), ST-40 ( Feng long ), Yin tang ( Ex ), LI-20 ( Ying xiang ), BL-2 ( Zhan zhu ), GB-20 ( Feng chi )

The accompanying points : ST-36 ( Zu san li ), K-7 ( Fu liu ), Bi tong ( Ex ), BL-12 ( Feng men ), LI-4 ( He gu ), GB-20 ( Feng chi ), K-3 ( Tai xi )

Bi tong is at the junction of the maxilla and the nasal cavity, near the upper end of the nasolabial groove and it opens the nose with LI-20. The pair of GV-23 and Yin tang eliminate the inflammation of sinuses and stops discharge from the sinuses. It is good to use moxibustion on GV-23 for chronic cases. ST-40 transforms the phlegm. Liv-2 clears the heat and reduces the Liv channel ( Liv channel problem usually causes sinusitis ). K-3 is for chronic case. BL-12 and GB-20 eliminate the wind. Strong manipulation is used.

### <85> Stuffy nose

There are many causes for this symptom. Medical consultation is essential. Usually external wind ( pathogen ) is related and there are allergy cases too. The prescription here is for symptoms only and the treatment of the causing diseases is necessary. The treatment idea is to open the orifice of nose and eliminate the wind from the head.

The main points : GB-20 ( Feng chi ), Lu-6 ( Kong zui ), GB-21 ( Jian jing ), GV-23 ( Shang xing ), BL-12 ( Feng men ), GV-14 ( Da zhui ), LI-4 ( He gu ), BL-67 ( Zhi yin ), LI-19 ( Kou he liao )

The accompanying points : GB-31 ( Feng shi ), LI-20 ( Ying xiang ), BL-10 ( Tian zhu ), LI-11 ( Qu chi ), Bi tong ( Ex ), Yin tang ( Ex ), Liv-2 ( Xing jian )

BL-12 eliminates the wind, GV-14 clears the heat, Lu-6 is the Xi cleft point of the lung. GB-20 eliminates the wind. BL-67 causes the Qi to descend and relieve the tension of nose. Bi tong is at the junction of the maxilla and the nasal cavity, near the upper end of the nasolabial groove and it opens the nose with LI-20. Liv-3 relieves the Qi stagnation of liver ( Liver channel is related with the problem of stuffy nose ). Strong manipulation is used.

### <86> Tinnitus – deficiency of Kidneys

Medical consultation is essential. In Traditional Chinese Medicine (TCM), if tinnitus decreases when pressing the ear, it is diagnosed as kidney deficiency. The patients can experience dizziness, weak lower limbs, weak waist and fatigue. The treatment idea is to tonify kidneys to nourish the orifice ( ears ).

The main points : GB-20 ( Feng chi ), SI-19 ( Ting gong ), SI-3 ( Hou xi ), BL-23 ( Shen shu ), GB-41 ( Zu lin qi ), GB-31 ( Feng shi ), TB-21 ( Er men ), TB-17 ( Yi feng ), GB-2 ( Ting hui ), TB-3 ( Zhong zhu ), CV-4 ( Guan yuan )

The accompanying points : SP-6 ( San yin jiao ), K-7 ( Fu liu ), GV-4 ( Ming men ), GB-43 ( Xia xi ), TB-5 ( Wai guan ), K-3 ( Tai xi ), Liv-3 ( Tai chong )

K-3, BL-23, CV-4, SP-6 and GV-4 tonify kidneys. SI-3 is the distant point for ear but it also tonifies kidneys. The local points of ear are used to regulate the Qi and blood around the ear. GB-43 clears the heat of GB channel. Considering the degree of deficiency, the number of needles is modified. Too many needles can make the situation worse. Soft manipulation is used for this case.

### <87> Tinnitus – liver fire

Medical consultation is essential. The liver fire attacking the orifices in the head can cause the tinnitus. The patient can experience emotional impatience, insomnia, bitter taste in the mouth, headache or pain on the area of rib bones. The treatment idea is to cool the heat and fire from the liver and regulate the ear and open the orifice.

The main points : SI-19 ( Ting gong ), Tai yang ( Ex ) : bloodletting technique, GB-20 ( Feng chi ), Liv-2 ( Xing jian ), GB-43 ( Xia xi ), GB-2 ( Ting hui ), TB-17 ( Yi feng ), TB-21 ( Er men ), TB-3 ( Zhong zhu ), GB-41 ( Zu lin qi ), Liv-3 ( Tai chong )

The accompanying points : BL-18 ( Gan shu ), Er jian ( Ex, auricular acupuncture ) : bloodletting technique, K-3 ( Tai xi ), BL-23 ( Shen shu ), GB-34 ( Yang ling quan ), BL-19 ( Dan shu )

Liv-2 and GB-43 clear the heat of Liv and GB channels. TB-3 is the distant point for the ear and GB-20 calms the wind from the liver. K-3 and BL-23 nourish the Kidneys to hold the liver fire and direct the Qi downwards. BL-18 and BL-19 nourish Liv and GB to calm the fire and prevent the deficiency of Yin. Strong manipulation is used.

### <88> Tinnitus – nervousness

Medical consultation is essential. This type of tinnitus is from emotional and mental instability. The heart generates the pathological fire and it causes tinnitus or the deficiency syndrome the orifice ( ear ) is not nourished. The patient experiences dizziness, emotional instability, insomnia or headache. The common causes are nervousness, neurosis, mental depression or hysteria. The treatment idea is to calm the mind and emotion, connect the heart and kidneys and control the heart. Depending on the excess syndrome or deficiency syndrome, you can modify the points or choose the manipulation methods.

The main points : K-3 ( Tai xi ), GB-20 ( Feng chi ), ST-8 ( Tou wei ), GV-20 ( Bai hui ), TB-2 ( Ye men ) to TB-3 ( Zhong zhu ), Ht-7 ( Shen men ), SI-19 ( Ting gong ), GV-26 ( Shui gou ), PC-8 ( Lao gong ), SI-3 ( Hou xi ), Liv-2 ( Xing jian ), Si shen cong ( Ex )

The accompanying points : CV-17 ( Shan zhong ), Liv-3 ( Tai chong ), An mian ( Ex ), GV-20 ( Bai hui ), SP-6 ( San yin jiao ), LI-4 ( He gu ), PC-6 ( Nei guan ) to TB-5 ( Wai guan )

An mian is at the middle point between GB-20 and TB-17 and treats insomnia and emotional instability. This prescription is the combination of points that calm the mind and connect the heart and kidneys. Deep needling from PC-6 to TB-5 generates strong stimulation on PC and TB-2 to TB-3 generates strong stimulation on TB channel. GV-26 opens the orifice of the patient. The accompanying points eliminate the Qi stagnation to control the emotion and calm the mind. The medium level manipulation is used.

## <89> Tonsillitis

This is the inflammation of the tonsils. Medical consultation is essential. The patient can experience sore throat, fever, swollen tonsils and the sensitive lymph nodes on the sides of the neck. The common causes are viral or bacterial infections. The treatment idea is to eliminate the heat form tonsils, ST and LI channels and eliminate the inflammation. The tonsils are related with the Yang ming channels ( ST and LI ) and Lu channel.

The main points : LI-4 ( He gu ), ST-44 ( Nei ting ), SP-6 ( San yin jiao ), Lu-11 ( Shao shang ), SI-17 ( Tian rong ), GB-21 ( Jian jing ), GV-14 ( Da zhui ), CV-22 ( Tian tu )

The accompanying points : LI-2 ( Er jian ), ST-45 ( Li Dui ), ST-36 ( Zu san li ), Er jian ( Ex., Auricular acupuncture ), LI-11 ( Qu chi ), Jing well points of the hands

Er jian ( Auricular acupuncture ) is the top of the ears. Bloodletting technique on Er jian will clear the heat from the head. LI-2 and ST-44 are the Xing spring points the clear the heat. Lu-11 and ST-45 are the Jing well points to clear the heat. LI-4, LI-11 and ST-36 clear the heat and infection. GV-14 clears the body heat and inflammation when strong manipulation is used.

# | 12 |

# Eyes

**<90> Cataract**

This is a clouding of the normally clear lens of the eye. It is related with old age. Medical consultation is essential. The symptoms are clouded vision, double vision in one eye, need for brighter light for reading and other activities, difficulty with night vision or frequent changes in eyeglass prescription. The treatment idea is to eliminate the ascending Yang of liver, Wind from liver, nourish Yin of kidneys and liver and activate the movement of Qi and blood around the eyes.

The main points : Tai yang ( Ex ) : bloodletting technique, TB-5 ( Wai guan ), GB-41 ( Zu lin qi ), GB-20 ( Feng chi ), BL-18 ( Gan shu ), GB-16 ( Mu chuang ), Liv-3 ( Tai chong ), ST-1 ( Cheng qi ), K-7 ( Fu liu ), BL-1 ( Jing Ming ), Qiu hou ( Ex ), GB-37 ( Guang ming )

The accompanying points : BL-7 ( Tong tian ), Liv-8 ( Qu quan ), Liv-2 ( Xing jian ), LI-4 ( He gu ), BL-23 ( Shen shu ), K-3 ( Tai xi ), SI-6 ( Yang lao ), K-7 ( Fu liu )

Qiu hou is the extra point under the eye located at the junction of the lateral one quarter and medial three quarters of the inferior border of the infra-orbital margin. Qiu hou activates the movement of Qi and blood around the eyes and treats the eye diseases. BL-1, ST-1 are local points of eyes. BL-7 activates the movement of Qi around head and eyes and nourishes the eyes. GB-37 is the special point to benefit the eyes. Liv-3 nourishes the liver and K-7 tonifies kidneys to nourish the liver. GB-20 eliminates the wind from liver. SI-6 is the Xi cleft point of SI and it is used to treat the blurred vision.

### <91> Conjunctivitis

This is an inflammation or infection of conjunctiva. The symptoms are irritating eyes and reddish eyes. Medical consultation is essential. This disease does not affect the vision much. The treatment idea is to clear the heat of the eyes, eliminate the inflammation. Clearing the liver heat and eliminating the wind is essential.

The main points : Liv-2 ( Xing jian ), Liv-1 ( Da dun ), ST-1 ( Cheng qi ), Tai yang ( Ex ) : bloodletting technique, GB-43 ( Xia xi ), BL-2 ( Zan zhu ), LI-4 ( He gu ), GB-20 ( Feng chi ), GB-1 ( Tong zi liao ), Er jian ( Ex., Auricular acupuncture ) : bloodletting technique

The accompanying points : SP-10 ( Xue hai ), Liv-3 ( Tai chong ), BL-1 ( Jing ming ), Liv-8 ( Qu quan ), K-3 ( Tai xi ), Yin tang ( Ex ), LI-1 ( Shang yang )

The local points ( BL-2, ST-1, Tai yang, Yin tang, BL-1 and GB-1 ) are used to activate the local movement of Qi and blood and clear the heat at the local area. Tai yang is at the lateral sides of the head. Liv-2, GB-43 clears the heat of Liv and GB channels. GB-20 eliminates the wind. LI-4 clears the heat and inflammation. Yin tang is at the middle point between the eyebrows. Liv-8 and K-3 nourish the liver and kidneys. LI-1 is the Jing well point that eliminates the heat and inflammation. Bloodletting technique is used for LI-1 and Liv-1

### <92> Electric ophthalmia, Arc flash ophthalmitis

This is caused by intensive and long exposure to gas welding, ultraviolet or motion-picture filming etc. Medical consultation is essential. The symptoms are edema in the conjunctiva, photophobia, hyperemia, tearing or eyelid spasm. The patient experience heat on eyes, eye tensions, the sensation of sands in the eyes. The treatment idea is to eliminate the heat and wind from the eyes

The main points : GB-43 ( Xia xi ), BL-2 ( Zan zhu ), Tai yang ( Ex ) : bloodletting technique, ST-2 ( Si bai ), Liv-2 ( Xing jian ), GB-20 ( Feng chi ), BL-1 ( Jing ming ), GB-37 ( Guang ming )
The accompanying points : LI-4 ( He gu ), Liv-3 ( Tai chong ), GB-31 ( Feng shi ), SI-6 ( Yang lao ), LI-11 ( Qu chi ), Yin tang ( Ex )

Tai yang is at the lateral sides of the head. Yin tang is at the middle point between the eyebrows. Tai yang and Yin tang are local points around the eyes. Liv-2 and GB-43 eliminate the heat from the eyes. The local points around the eyes clears the heat and inflammation of the eyes. GB-20 eliminates the wind. GB-37 is the special point to benefit the eyes. SI-6 is the Xi cleft point of SI and benefits the eyes. LI-4 and LI-11 clears the heat and inflammation. Strong manipulation is used to eliminate the heat from the eyes.

### <93> Eye pain

There are many causes and it is complicated to specify one cause for this symptom. Medical consultation is essential. In TCM the eye pain is stagnation of Qi and blood or heat and inflammation in the eyes.

The main points : Liv-3 ( Tai chong ), GB-41 ( Zu lin qi ), ST-2 ( Si bai ), GB-14 ( Yang bai ), LI-4 ( He gu ), Ba xie ( Ex ), GB-16 ( Mu chuang ), Ht-8 ( Shao fu ) : reducing method, GB-20 ( Feng chi ), Tai yang ( Ex ) : bloodletting technique
The accompanying points : GB-37 ( Guang ming ), Liv-2 ( Xing jian ), BL-1 ( Jing ming ), Yin tang ( Ex ), GB-31 ( Feng shi ), TB-23 ( Si zhu kong ), GB-34 ( Yang ling quan )

GB-20 and Liv-3 regulate the Qi and blood around the eyes and relieve the pain. The local points around the eyes relieve the pain. Ba xie is proximal to the margins of the webs between all five fingers at the junction of the red and white skin on the dorsal side of the hand. Total 8 points on both sides. Ba xie ( 8 points ) is the special point for eye pain. LI-4 is for the problem of head. Tai yang is at the lateral sides of the head. Yin tang is at the middle point of the eyebrows. GB-34 relieves the tension and the pains. GB-37 is the special point for the eyes. Strong manipulation is used.

### <94> Glaucoma

The high pressure inside the eyes damages the optic nerves that connect the eyes and the brain. Medical consultation is essential. This disease can lead to loss of vision if not properly treated early. The patients experience vomiting, nausea, headache, intense eye pain, red eye, blurred vision or vision of rings around the lights etc. The treatment idea is to eliminate the tension in the eyes, eliminate the wind, pacify the liver yang, eliminate the liver heat, nourish liver Yin and kidneys.

The main points : ST-36 ( Zu san li ), LI-4 ( He gu ), Liv-2 ( Xing jian ), BL-2 ( Zan zhu ), GB-1 ( Tong zi liao ), GB-20 ( Feng chi ), SP-6 ( San yin jiao ), K-3 ( Tai xi ), BL-18 ( Gan shu ), Tai yang ( Ex ) : bloodletting technique, GB-37 ( Guang ming )

The accompanying points : BL-62 ( Shen mai ), GB-31 ( Feng shi ), BL-63 ( Jin men ), Liv-3 ( Tai chong ), K-7 ( Fu liu ), GB-41 ( Xia xi ), LI-11 ( Qu chi )

Tai yang is at the lateral sides of the head. This point eliminates the heat around the head and eyes. The local points around the eyes can eliminate the heat, tension and move Qi and blood. Liv-2 and GB-41 clear the heat of Liv and GB channels to clear the heat in the eyes. GB-20 eliminates the liver wind. SP-6 and BL-18 nourish liver. K-3 nourish kidneys. BL-63 and BL-62 benefit the eyes. K-7 ad Liv-3 nourish kidneys and liver. Strong manipulation is used around the eyes and the points that eliminate the wind, heat or liver yang.

### <95> Night blindness, Nyctalopia

Liver disease, vitamin A deficiency, diabetes, cataract or glaucoma etc can cause this symptom. Medical consultation is essential. Treatment of the causing disease is necessary. The treatment idea here is to nourish the liver to nourish the eyes.

The main points : ST-1 ( Cheng qi ), BL-23 ( Shen shu ), BL-18 ( Gan shu ), TB-23 ( Si zhu kong ), BL-1 ( Jing ming ), LI-4 ( He gu ), BL-2 ( Zan zhu ), K-7 ( Fu liu ), Liv-3 ( Tai chong )

The accompanying points : GB-16 ( Mu chuang ), TB-22 ( He liao ), SI-3 ( Hou xi ), GB-3 ( Shang guan ), LI-11 ( Qu chi ), ST-36 ( Zu san li ), GB-37 ( Guang ming ), Liv-8 ( Qu quan )

The local points around the eyes move Qi and blood to nourish the eyes. Liv-8 and Kid-7 nourish the liver and kidneys. SI-3 opens the GV channel and tonifies kidneys. ST-36 tonifies Qi. GB-37 benefits the eyes. BL-23 and BL-18 tonify kidneys and liver. Medium level manipulation is used.

### <96> Ocular fatigue, Asthenopia

The main causes are focusing on a book, cell phone, TV or monitor without stopping and it make the ciliary muscles and the extraocular muscles strained. Medical consultation is essential. The symptoms are eyes fatigue, sore eyes, difficulty in refocusing, blurred vision, dryness on eyes, headache, sensitivity to bright lights, discomfort in eyes, irritated eyes or burning eyes. The treatment idea is to eliminate the strain on the eyes, activate the movement of Qi and blood around the eyes using the local points, nourish the liver and kidneys to recover from the ocular fatigue.

The main points : GB-1 ( Tong zi liao ), SP-10 ( Xue hai ), GB-20 ( Feng chi ), SI-3 ( Hou xi ), LI-4 ( He gu ), Liv-3 ( Tai chong ), BL-10

( Tian zhu ), K-3 ( Tai xi ), BL-18 ( Gan shu ), GV-12 ( Shen zhu ), GB-16 ( Mu chuang )

The accompanying points : K-7 ( Fu liu ), Liv-2 ( Xing jian ), SP-6 ( San yin jiao ), BL-23 ( Shen shu ), SI-6 ( Yang lao ), ST-36 ( Zu san li ), GB-34 ( Yang ling quan ), TB-3 ( Zhong zhu ), GB-37 ( Guang ming )

GB-20 is the special point to regulate the Qi and blood of head including eyes. It relieves the eye strain. TB-3 activates the TB channel to recover from fatigue. GB-37 is the special point to benefit the vision. The local points around the eyes are used. SI-3 tonifies kidneys to nourish the eyes. Liv-3 and Liv-2 eliminate the heat and strain on eyes. GV-12 tonifies the Qi. K-3 and K-7 tonify kidneys to nourish eyes. BL-18 and BL-23 nourish liver and kidneys. Medium level manipulation is used. The moxibustion can be used for the distant points

### <97> Presbyopia, Eyesight of the aged

Aging process causes this symptom. Medical consultation is essential. The treatment idea is activating the Qi and blood around the eyes, nourish liver and kidneys to clarify the vision.

The main points : Da gu kong ( Ex ), SI-6 ( Yang lao ), GV-12 ( Shen zhu ), Liv-8 ( Qu quan ), GB-20 ( Feng chi ), Xiao gu kong ( Ex ), Liv-3 ( Tai chong ), GB-37 ( Guang ming ), ST-36 ( Zu san li ), BL-23 ( Shen shu )

The accompanying points : SP-10 ( Xue hai ), GV-16 ( Feng fu ), BL-18 ( Gan shu ), GB-21 ( Jian jing ), LI-4 ( He gu ), CV-4 ( Guan yuan ), K-7 ( Fu liu ), SP-6 ( San yin jiao ), TB-22 ( He liao ), LI-10 ( Shou san li )

Da gu kong is at the center of the joint between the distal and middle phalanges on the dorsal side of the thumb. Xiao gu kong is at the center of the joint between the distal and middle phalanges on the dorsal side of the little finger. Da gu kong and Xiao gu kong benefit the eyes and calm the rebellious Qi. GB-21 regulates the Qi. Liv-8 nourishes liver. GB-37 is the special point to benefit the eyes. SI-6 is the Xi cleft point of SI and it benefits the eyes. GV-12 tonifies lung and increases the Qi. Liv-3, SP-6, CV-4, K-7, BL-18 and BL-23 tonify and nourish kidneys and liver. GV-16 and GB-20 eliminate the wind from the head. Moxibustion on the distant points and needling on the head are more effective than just needling.

### <98> Ptosis, drooping of the upper eyelids.

This is a symptom of drooping of the upper eyelids. Medical consultation is essential. The cause is dysfunction of the muscles that raise the eyelid or their nerves. The treatment idea is activating the Qi and blood in the upper eyelids, tonify spleen and stomach. The upper eyelids correspond to stomach and the lower eyelids to spleen in TCM diagnosis. And the spleen and stomach are responsible for the weak muscle.

The main points : GB-20 ( Feng chi ), LI-4 ( He gu ), SP-9 ( Yin ling quan ), Yu yao ( Ex ), BL-4 ( Qu cha ), BL-21 ( Wei shu ), GB-1 ( Tong zi liao ), Liv-3 ( Tai chong ), GB-34 ( Yang ling quan ), BL-62 ( Shen mai ), BL-2 ( Zan zhu )

The accompanying points : BL-20 ( Pi shu ), GB-14 ( Yang bai ), ST-43 ( Xian gu ), ST-36 ( Zu san li ), K-6 ( Zhao hai ), TB-23 ( Si zhu kong ), ST-2 ( Si bai )

Yu yao is at the middle of eyebrows, directly above the pupil. The local points around the eyes are mainly used for this case to activate the Qi and blood to recover. ST-36 and SP-9 tonify spleen and stomach to nourish the eyelids. K-6 and BL-62 open the extraordinary channels of Yin heel vessel ( Yin qiao mai ) and Yang heel vessel ( Yang qiao mai ) that control the opening and closing the eyes. GB-34 and Liv-3 nourish the liver. Soft manipulation is used.

### <99> Spasm of eyelid, Blepharospasm

This is an abnormal contraction of the eyelid muscles. Medical consultation is essential. The clear cause is not known but they guess the abnormal brain function in the part of the brain that controls muscles can be the reason. Symptoms can be triggered by mental stress, fatigue, neurological conditions like Tourette syndrome or Parkinson's disease. The symptoms of movements are wind and the wind is generated from liver in TCM. The treatment idea is to pacify the wind, regulate the Qi and blood around the eyes to relieve the tension, eliminate the heat and calm the brain and mind.

The main points : BL-62 ( Shen mai ), GB-3 ( Shang guan ), GB-31 ( Feng shi ), GB-14 ( Yang bai ), K-6 ( Zhao hai ), GB-1 ( Tong zi liao ), GB-20 ( Feng chi ), Liv-3 ( Tai chong ), BL-2 ( Zan zhu ), ST-2 ( Si bai )

The accompanying points : GB-34 ( Yang ling quan ), Liv-2 ( Xing jiang ), TB-17 ( Yi feng ), GB-21 ( Jian jing ), GB-34 ( Yang ling quan ), LI-11 ( Qu chi ), PC-6 ( Nei guan ), LI-4 ( He gu ), GV-20 ( Bai hui )

The local points activate the Qi and blood to relieve the tension around the eyes. GB-20, TB-17, GV-20, Liv-3 and GB-34 eliminate the wind. K-6 and BL-62 regulate the movement of eyelids. Strong manipulation is used.

**<100> Stye**
The cause is external infection. Medical consultation is essential. The treatment idea is to clear the heat of the inflammation, move Qi and blood around the eyes to recover rapidly.

The main points : ST-44 ( Nei ting ), Ht-8 ( Shao fu ) : reducing method, GB-14 ( Yang bai ), Liv-2 ( Xing jian ), LI-11 ( Qu chi ), GB-20 ( Feng chi ), Tai yang ( Ex ) : bloodletting technique, ST-1 ( Cheng qi ), Da gu kong ( Ex )

The accompanying points : GB-43 ( Xia xi ), LI-4 ( He gu ), SI-6 ( Yang lao ), BL-2 ( Zan zhu ), GB-37 ( Guang ming ), LI-3 ( San jian ), Jian ming ( Ex )

Da gu kong is at the dorsal side of the thumb, at the midpoint of the proximal interphalangeal joint. Jian ming is inside the inferior margin of the orbit of eyes, about 0.4 cun from the BL-1. The local points move Qi and blood around the eyes, clear the heat from the local inflammation. Da gu kong clears the heat from the eyes. ST-44, LI-11 and LI-4 clear the heat of the inflammation. Liv-3 clears the heat of liver. Jian ming is the local point to clear the heat. Strong manipulation is used. Moxibustion can be used on Da gu kong.

### <101> Watery eyes ( excessive tearing ), Epiphora

This is too much tear in the eyes and that makes the watering eyes. Medical consultation is essential. The causes are various including problems in the eyes, liver diseases or reduced tear outflow. The treatment of the causing diseases is necessary. Reduced tear outflow is from the obstruction at any portion of the nasolacrimal drainage system. In that case, eliminating the obstruction is necessary. The treatment prescription here does not include the obstruction problem. The treatment idea is to eliminate the excessive sensitivity of the eyes, eliminate the heat from the eyes, increase the Qi to protect the eyes from the wind, regulate the Qi and blood around the eyes.

The main points : BL-1 ( Jing ming ), GB-43 ( Xia xi ), Liv-2 ( Xing jian ), ST-36 ( Zu san li ), LI-4 ( He gu ), GV-23 ( Shang xing ), ST-1 ( Cheng qi ), Tai yang ( Ex ) : bloodletting technique, Yin tang ( Ex ), GB-20 ( Feng chi )

The accompanying points : BL-2 ( Zan zhu ), ST-10 ( Xue hai ), Qiu hou ( Ex ), SI-6 ( Yang lao ), GV-16 ( Feng fu ), LI-10 ( Shou san li ), GB-31 ( Feng shi )

Tai yang is at the lateral sides of the head. Yin tang is at the middle point of the eyebrows. It eliminates the heat and regulates the local Qi and blood when used with GV-23. GB-20 eliminates the wind. BL-1, BL-2, ST-1 and Tai yang eliminate the local heat from the eyes and reduce the sensitivity. ST-36 tonifies Qi to protect the eyes from the external wind that may be the cause of tear. SI-6 is the Xi cleft point of SI channel to benefit the eyes. Qiu hou is at the junction of the medial 3/4 and the lateral 1/4 of the infraorbital margin. Qiu hou regulates the Qi and blood of the eyes. Soft manipulation is used.

# | 13 |

# Infection, fever

**<102> Cold (1)**
This is common cold. Infection happens by virus. Everyone can be infected every year. Medical consultation is essential. The treatment idea is to activate the immune system, eliminate the wind pathogen, clear the heat ( in case of wind heat pathogen ), eliminate the phlegm and open the orifice ( nose ).

The main points : GV-14 ( Da zhui ), ST-36 ( Zu san li ), GB-20 ( Feng chi ), TB-5 ( Wai guan ), LI-11 ( Qu chi ), BL-12 ( Feng men ), LI-20 ( Ying xiang ), Lu-7 ( Lie que ), San shang ( Ex ), LI-4 ( He gu )
The accompanying points : BL-13 ( Fei shu ), Bi tong ( Ex ), CV-22 ( Tian tu ), ST-40 ( Feng long ), Yin tang ( Ex ), K-6 ( Zhao hai ), GV-4 ( Ming men ) : in case of coldness.

There are heat syndrome and cold syndrome. Depending on the pattern diagnosis, the point selection can be made. Lu-7 and K-6 are the combination to eliminate coughing and benefit the throat. LI-11 and LI-4 eliminate the fever. GV-14 clears the heat by strong manipulation in case of wind heat pathogen. San huang is a group of three points near the upper region of thumb nail. San shang eliminates the fever of cold. TB-5 liberates the external layer to eliminate the pathogen. BL-12 and GB-20 eliminate the wind. Yin tang is at the middle point between the eyebrows. Bi tong is at the highest point of the nasolabial groove. LI-20, Yin tang and Bi tong open the nose. ST-36 tonifies the Qi if manipulated in tonifying method to increase the immune power. ST-40 eliminates the phlegm. Strong manipulation is used to eliminate the pathogen.

### <103> Cold (2) – heat type with unclear consciousness.

This is the common cold of heat type with unclear consciousness. Medical consultation is essential. The treatment idea is to open the orifice to make the consciousness clear, eliminate the heat and fever.

The main points : LI-4 ( He gu ), GV-14 ( Da zhui ), San shang ( Ex ), LI-11 ( Qu chi ), Shi xuan ( Ex ), Ht-8 ( Shao fu ) : reducing method, GV-26 ( Shui gou ), Ren zhong xin ( Ex ), ST-44 ( Nei ting )

The accompanying points : PC-6 ( Nei guan ), GV-20 ( Bai hui ), Er jian ( Auricular point ) : bloodletting technique, Lu-10 ( Yu ji ), LI-1 ( Shang yang ) : bloodletting technique

Shi xuan is at the tips of the fingers. San huang is a group of three points near the upper region of thumb nail. San shang eliminates the fever of cold. Ren zhong xin is at the middle of the middle phalanges at the palmar side of the finger. It clears the heat. Er jian is the point of auricular acupuncture. Bloodletting technique is used for LI-1, San shang and Er jian. LI-1, Lu-10, ST-44, LI-4 and LI-11 clears the heat. Shi xuan, GV-26 and PC-6 open the orifice. The strong manipulation is used to eliminate the heat pathogen and open the orifice.

### <104> Fever

This is about the body heat for some reason. Body heat is the expression of pathogen or internal problem. Medical consultation is essential. Treatment of the causing disease is necessary. These points can be used to drop the body heat. It is not necessary to use all of these points. You can choose 3-4 points that you think the most proper for the case. The treatment idea is to clear the heat.

The points : Lu-5 ( Chi ze ), Liv-2 ( Xing jian ), Jing well points of the hands and feet : bloodletting technique, LI-2 ( Er jian ), ST-37 ( Shang ju xu ), LI-4 ( He gu ), Er jian ( Auricular acupuncture point ) : bloodletting technique, LI-11 ( Qu chi ), GV-14 ( Da zhui ), SP-6 ( San yin jiao ), The veins on the back of the ear ( Auricular acupuncture points ) : bloodletting technique, Shi xuan ( Ex ) : bloodletting technique

All of these points have the function of cooling the body. Shi xuan is at the tips of the finger. Er jian is at the top of the ear. Bloodletting technique is used for Shi xuan, Er jian, Jing well points and the 3 veins on the back of the ear. Strong manipulation is used for all other points.

### <105> Influenza, the flu (1)

This is an infectious disease caused by influenza viruses. The symptoms are fever, sore throat, low appetite, weak body, coughing, runny nose, headache, fatigue and muscle pain. Medical consultation is essential. The symptoms can be severe or mild depending on the cases. The treatment idea is to clear the heat pathogen and wind, regulate the lung and stop coughing, open the orifice ( nose ) and regulate the digestion

The main points : Lu-7 ( Lie que ), GB-20 ( Feng chi ), SP-6 ( San yin jiao ), LI-11 ( Qu chi ), Lu-5 ( Chi ze ), LI-1 ( Shang yang ), Lu-10 ( Yu ji ), LI-4 ( He gu ), GV-14 ( Da zhui )

The accompanying points : BL-13 ( Fei shu ), TB-5 ( Wai guan ), Yin tang ( Ex ), K-3 ( Tai xi ), K-6 ( Zhao hai ), ST-36 ( Zu san li ), LI-20 ( Ying xiang ), CV-22 ( Tian tu ), PC-6 ( Nei guan ), Shi xuan ( Ex ), Bi tong ( Ex )

Lu-5 reduces the excess heat of lung. LI-1, LI-4, LI-11, Lu-10 and GV-14 eliminate the heat pathogen. K-6 and Lu-7 benefit the throat and stop coughing. K-3 prevents the body from being dried. CV-22 eliminates the phlegm and stops coughing. Yin tang and LI-20 open the nose. Bloodletting technique is used on LI-1. If the fever is severe, bloodletting technique is used on Shi xuan or Jing well points. Shi xuan is at the tips of the fingers.

### <106> Influenza, the flu (2)

This is an infectious disease caused by influenza viruses. The symptoms are fever, sore throat, low appetite, weak body, coughing, runny nose, headache, fatigue and muscle pain. Medical consultation is essential. The symptoms can be severe or mild depending on the cases. The treatment idea is to clear the heat pathogen and wind, regulate the lung and stop coughing, open the orifice ( nose ) and regulate the digestion

The main points : GV-20 ( Bai hui ), San shang ( Ex ), LI-4 ( He gu ), LI-11 ( Qu chi ),
The accompanying points : SP-6 ( San yin jiao ), ST-36 ( Zu san li ), Ren zhong xin ( Ex ), GV-26 ( Shui gou )

### <107> Malaria

Malaria is an infectious disease from mosquitos. It affects humans and other vertebrates. Medical consultation is essential. The typical symptoms include fever, vomiting, headache, fatigue. It can cause seizures, coma, jaundice or even death. The main treatment idea is clear the heat from the Shao yang region and Yang ming region depending on the TCM diagnosis syndromes.

The main points : PC-5 (Jian shi ), GB-40 ( Qiu xu ), GV-9 ( Zhi yang ), Nue men ( Ex ), GV-14 ( Da zhui ), LI-11 ( Qu chi ), GB-41 ( Zu lin qi ), LI-4 ( He gu )
The accompanying points : SP-6 ( San yin jiao ), GV-26 ( Shui gou ), PC-6 ( Nei guan ), ST-36 ( Zu san li ), Jing well points of hands : bloodletting technique

Nue men is the extra acupoint for malaria. This point is Located on the back of the hand, in front of the third and fourth metacarpophalangeal joints, slightly posterior to the webbing between the middle finger and ring finger, at the junction of the red and white skin, with a total of 2 points on each hand.

### <108> Mumps, epidemic parotitis

Mumps is an inflammation of parotid salivary glands. The symptoms are tenderness, pain and swelling in the cheek and jaw area. Medical consultation is essential. The main treatment idea is to eliminate the inflammation and relieve the local pain. The local acupoints and the treatment of inflammation is used.

The main points : LI-11 ( Qu chi ), ST-44 ( Nei ting ), ST-36 ( Zu san li ), TB-17 ( Yi feng ), ST-6 ( Jia che ), LI-4 ( He gu ), Liv-2 ( Xing jian ), Tai yang ( Ex ) : bloodletting technique

The accompanying points : Liv-3 ( Tai chong ), SP-10 ( Xue hai ), Lu-10 ( Yu ji ), SP-6 ( San yin jiao ), Lu-11 ( Shao shang ), LI-1 ( Shang yang ) : bloodletting technique, Liv-8 ( Qu quan )

### <109> Shingles, Herpes Zoster (1) – on the face

The chickenpox virus ( varicella zoster virus ) stays dormant in the body and it causes shingles when reactivated. Medical consultation is essential. The skin rash can appear on the face, chest, abdomen or lateral sides of the thorax. The prescription here is for the rashes on the face. The treatment idea is to clear the heat and wind, eliminate the toxins of the virus and regulate the Qi and blood of the face to eliminate the pain and rashes from the face.

The main points : ST-36 ( Zu san li ), ST-44 ( Nei ting ), LI-2 ( Er jian ), BL-10 ( Tian zhu ), GB-20 ( Feng chi ), Liv-2 ( Xing jian ), GV-12 ( Shen zhu ), GB-43 ( Xia xi ), LI-11 ( Qu chi ), Tai yang ( Ex ) : bloodletting technique, LI-4 ( He gu ), Er jian ( Auricular acupuncture point ) : bloodletting technique, GB-31 ( Feng shi )

The accompanying points : BL-13 ( Fei shu ), TB-17 ( Yi feng ), SI-3 ( Hou xi ), Jing well points of the hands and feet, TB-5 ( Wai guan ), Ashi points where has pain.

Er jian is the auricular acupuncture point and is at the top of the ear. Er jian, LI-11, LI-4, Jing well points, ST-44 and LI-2 eliminate the heat. LI-4 and LI-11 eliminate the heat toxins. Tai yang is at the lateral sides of the head and it eliminates the heat from the face. TB-5 liberates the exterior layer to eliminate the pathogen. The strong manipulation is used. Bloodletting technique is used for Er jian, Tai yang and Jing well points.

**<110> Shingles, Herpes Zoster (2) – on the chest, abdomen or lateral sides.**

The chickenpox virus ( varicella zoster virus ) stays dormant in the body and it causes shingles when reactivated. Medical consultation is essential. The skin rash can appear on the face, chest, abdomen or lateral sides of the thorax. The prescription here is for the rashes on the chest, abdomen or lateral sides of the thorax. The treatment idea is to clear the heat and wind, eliminate the toxins of the virus and regulate the Qi and blood to eliminate the pain and rashes.

The main points : Ashi points, GV-14 ( Da zhui ), Liv-13 ( Zhang men ), SP-21 ( Da bao ), GB-34 ( Yang ling quan ), SP-15 ( Da heng ), LI-4 ( He gu ), Liv-2 ( Xing jian ), TB-5 ( Wai guan ), GB-24 ( Ri yue ), GB-43 ( Xia xi ), GB-40 ( Qiu xu ), GB-41 ( Zu lin qi )

The accompanying points : SP-9 ( Yin ling quan ), TB-6 ( Zhi gou ), ST-44 ( Nei ting ), PC-6 ( Nei guan ), ST-40 ( Feng long ), CV-12 ( Zhong wan ), LI- 11 ( Qu chi ), CV-4 ( Guan yuan ), BL-19 ( Dan shu ), BL-18 ( Gan shu )

The local points of the chest ( CV-17 ), abdomen ( CV-12, CV-4 ), lateral sides of the thorax ( SP-15 ) and GB-24, SP-21, Liv-13 are used to eliminate the local pain and toxins. The pathogen of shingles has the tendency to enter the ST, LI, Liv and GB channels. Usually heat and dampness attack the body. The prescription is to eliminate the heat toxins from the Liv, GB, ST, and LI channels and eliminate the dampness. Strong manipulation is used.

### <111> Tetanus, lockjaw

The cause is the bacterium toxin that makes the nervous system infected. Medical consultation is essential. The symptoms are muscle contractions of jaw and neck muscles, possible high fever, whole body paralysis, convulsions, spasm, paralysis with smiling face. This disease is life threatening. The treatment idea in acupuncture is to eliminate the wind, heat and inflammation, relieve the tension on the jaw and the whole body to stop spasm.

The main points : GB-20 ( Feng chi ), GV-14 ( Da zhui ), GB-34 ( Yang ling quan ), SI-3 ( Hou xi ), GV-26 ( Shui gou ), GB-34 ( Yang ling quan ), Liv-3 ( Tai chong ), ST-7 ( Xia guan ), GV-15 ( Ya men )

The accompanying points : LI-4 ( He gu ), GV-8 ( Jin suo ), PC-6 ( Nei guan ), LI-11 ( Qu chi ), GV-3 ( Yao yang guan ), BL-18 ( Gan shu ), BL-21 ( Wei shu ), BL-62 ( Shen mai )

GB-34, Liv-3 and B-18 relieve the muscle tensions. ST-7 is the local point to relieve the tension of jaw. GB-20 eliminates the wind to removes the convulsion and spasm. GV-15, GV-14 calm the nerve system and clear the heat in the nerves. SI-3 opens the channel of GV and stop the spasm and brain problems. LI-4 and LI-11 eliminate the heat and infection. Strong manipulation is used to eliminate the heat and infection. Electric acupuncture can be used to maintain the stimulation.

# | 14 |
# Women's health

**<112> Adnexitis, inflammation of the uterine appendages**

This is about the inflammation of the uterine appendages like fallopian tubes ( salpingitis ), the supporting ligaments ( parametritis ) or the ovaries ( oophoritis ). Medical consultation is essential. The main cause is bacterial infections like chlamydia, gonorrhea or a mixed infection of different bacteria. The acute inflammation causes lower abdominal pain, constipation, uterine bleeding or fever. The chronic inflammation causes irregular menstruation, pain or bleeding. The treatment idea is to eliminate the inflammation on the local area, activate the functions of the uterine appendages by unblocking the gynecology channels.

The main points : K-6 ( Zhao hai ), GB-34 ( Yang ling quan ), SP-6 ( Yin ling quan ), CV-3 ( Zhong ji ), GB-26 ( Dai mai ), ST-28 ( Shui dao ), Liv-3 ( Tai chong ), Lu-7 ( Lie que ), Ashi

The accompanying points : SP-10 ( Xue hai ), GV-4 ( Ming men ), BL-52 ( Zhi shi ), ST-27 ( Da ju ), BL-18 ( Gan shu ), K-7 ( Fu liu ), BL-32 ( Ci liao ), BL-23 ( Shen shu ), CV-4 ( Guan yuan )

The prescription is the combination of local points and the distant points. Lu-7 activates the CV channel to treat the Gynecology problems. Liv-3 and SP-6 activate the uterine functions. Ashi eliminates the local stagnation of Qi and inflammation. CV-4 tonifies the liver and kidneys. BL-23, BL-18 and BL-52 tonify kidneys. BL-32 eliminates the local inflammation. The strong manipulation is used for the acute inflammation. The moxibustion is used for the chronic situation.

### <113> Agalactia, Low breast milk supply

The milk is not generated much after the baby is born or the color of milk is too thin. Medical consultation is essential. In TCM, the causes are mainly deficiency problem of the mother. When the baby was born, if the mother lost too much blood, the mother can be in a deficiency state and is not able to generate sufficient milk. The ST channel is used frequently for this problem. The tonifying or nourishing method is used.

The main points : TB-4 ( Yang chi ), ST-36 ( Zu san li ), SI-1 ( Shao ze ), SP-6 ( San yin jiao ), CV-17 ( Shan zhong ) to the directions of breasts, GB-21 ( Jian jing ), CV-4 ( Guan yuan ), ST-18 ( Ru gen )

The accompanying points : K-7 ( Fu liu ), GB-12 ( Wan gu ), SP-10 ( Xue hai ), SI-11 ( Tian zong ), PC-6 ( Nei guan ), Liv-3 ( Tai chong )

SI-1 is the special point for low breast milk supply. CV-4, SP-10, ST-36 and SP-6 tonify the body. CV-17 can be needled by two needles that direct to the breasts. The local points near breasts promote or activate the function of breasts. Soft manipulation is used. Moxibustion is used on ST-18 to activate the breasts.

### <114> Amenorrhea (1)

There are many causes like hormone problems, emotional problems, mental stress, nutritional problems etc. Medical consultation is essential. In TCM, usually the treatment idea is regulating CV, Chong mai ( penetrating vessel ), Liv channel etc. The usual prescription is comprised of regulating CV, Chong mai, Liv and local points to stimulate ovaries. In case of overweight problem, weight loss treatment is very important because body phlegm can cause Amenorrhea. In case of emotional stress, relieving Liv channel and eliminating the heat is important. In case of deficiency, it is necessary to nourish the body.

The main points : K-6 ( Zhao hai ), ST-28 ( Shui dao ), SP-6 ( San yin jiao ), BL-23 ( Shen shu ), SP-10 ( Xue hai ), SP-4 ( Gong sun ), Liv-3 ( Tai chong ), SP-8 ( Di ji ), CV-7 ( Yin jiao ), SI-3 ( Hou xi )
The accompanying points : Liv-2 ( Xing jian ), Ht-7 ( Shen men ), BL-32 ( Ci liao ), BL-17 ( Ge shu ), Zi gong ( Ex ), Liv-8 ( Qu quan ), CV-6 ( Qi hai ), Lu-7 ( Lie que ), LI-4 ( He gu ), GV-4 ( Ming men ),

Regulate the Liv channels and open the Chong mai by SP-4. Open the CV channel by Lu-7. Zi gong is the extra point for regulating ovaries action. Medium level manipulation is used. The treatment is done everyday or once for 2 days. In case of deficiency or cold syndrome, the moxibustion can be used.

### <115> Amenorrhea (2)

There are many causes like hormone problems, emotional problems, mental stress, nutritional problems etc. Medical consultation is essential. In TCM, usually treat Amenorrhea regulating CV, Chong mai ( penetrating vessel ), Liv channel etc. The usual prescription is comprised of regulating CV, Chong mai, Liv and local points to stimulate ovaries. In case of overweight problem, weight loss treatment is very important because body phlegm can cause Amenorrhea. In case of emotional stress, relieving Liv channel and eliminating the heat is important. In case of deficiency, it is necessary to nourish the body.

The main points : LI-4 ( He gu ), SP-10 ( Xue hai ), GV-20 ( Bai hui ), GV-4 ( Ming men ), SP-4 ( Gong sun ), CV-7 ( Yin jiao ), SP-6 ( San yin jiao ), Zi gong ( Ex )

The accompanying points : PC-6 ( Nei guan ), ST-30 ( Qi chong ), SP-8 ( Di ji ), BL-23 ( Shen shu ), CV-4 ( Guan yuan ), BL-17 ( Ge shu )

Medium level manipulation is used. SP-4 opens Chong mai ( penetrating vessel ) and GV-4 and CV-4 activate the Kidneys Yang to strengthen the inferior burner. ST-40 ( Feng long ) can be added to eliminate the phlegm in case it is necessary.

### <116> Dysfunctional uterine bleeding ( DUB )

In TCM, this disease is called Beng lou. Medical consultation is essential. This disease is mainly related with CV channel, Chong mai ( penetrating vessel ) or Liv channel. There are many causes like emotional stress, nutritional imbalance etc. In TCM, the internal heat, deficiency of kidneys, blood, Qi of Spleen are the causes. Regulating CV channel, Chong mai, Liv channel and SP channel are the main principle of treatment.

The main points : Liv-1 ( Da dun ), SP-6 ( San yin jiao ), SP-1 ( Yin bai ), BL-20 ( Pi shu ), CV-7 ( Yin jiao ), SP-10 ( Xue hai ), SP-4 ( Gong sun ), Ht-7 ( Shen men )

The accompanying points : GV-20 ( Bai hui ), BL-40 ( Wei zhong ), GV-4 ( Ming men ), Lu-7 ( Lie que ), BL-18 ( Gan shu ), Liv-8 ( Qu quan ), CV-4 ( Guan yuan )

The Jing well points like SP-1 and Liv-1 are used to stop bleeding. SP-4 opens the Chong mai ( penetrating vessel ) and Lu-7 opens the CV channel. Medium level manipulation or moxibustion is used.

### <117> Excessive menstruation

The quantity of blood is excessive or the cycle is too short. Medical consultation is essential. In TCM, deficiency of spleen Qi can cause bleeding problem, malfunction of Liv channel, Chong mai ( penetrating vessel ), CV channel, or internal heat can cause this problem. The patient has to check the medical examination early because in occidental medicine there can have many causes like uterine cancer, bad blood circulation in pelvis, hormone problems etc.

The main points : SP-4 ( Gong sun ), SP-1 ( Yin bai ), LI-11 ( Qu chi ), GV-14 ( Da zhui ), CV-4 ( Guan yuan ), Liv-1 ( Da dun ), K-10 ( Yin gu ), SP-6 ( San yin jiao ), BL-27 ( Xiao chang shu ), ST-36 ( Zu san li )

The accompanying points : GV-20 ( Bai hui ), Liv-3 ( Tai chong ), K-3 ( Tai xi ), BL-32 ( Ci liao ), ST-27 ( Da ju ), BL-23 ( Shen shu ), Lu-5 ( Chi ze ), SP-10 ( Xue hai ), LI-4 ( He gu ), BL-17 ( Ge shu )

Jing well points like Liv-1 and SP-1 are used to stop bleeding. SP-10 and BL-17 are the special point to regulate the blood. In case of internal heat, reducing method is used to eliminate the heat. LI-11 (reducing) and GV-14 (reducing) can be added to clear the heat in case of internal heat. In case of deficiency or chronic cases, soft manipulation is used. Moxibustion is used for cold syndrome.

### <118> Excessive vaginal discharge

There are many causes like endometritis, cervicitis, weak constitution or tumor. Medical consultation is essential. The medical examination is necessary to prevent delaying treatment. In TCM, this symptom is considered as dampness and heat, coldness and dampness or deficiency of spleen qi etc. The main treatment principle is to eliminate the dampness and treat the syndromes.

The main points : SP-9 ( Yin ling quan ), GB-26 ( Dai mai ), GB-41 ( Zu lin qi ), Zi gong ( Ex ), SP-6 ( San yin jiao ), CV-6 ( Qi hai ), TB-6 ( Zhi gou )

The accompanying points : CV-3 ( Zhong ji ), ST-30 ( Qi chong ), ST-36 ( Zu san li ), CV-3 ( Zhong ji ), SP-10 ( Xue hai )

In case of coldness : use moxibustion on CV-4 ( Guan yuan ), CV-8 ( Shen que ), GV-4 ( Ming men )

In case of heat : add LI-2 ( Er jian ), GV-14 ( Da zhui ), Liv-2 ( Xing jian ), ST-44 ( Nei ting ), LI-11 ( Qu chi )

GB-41 is used to activate the Dai mai ( Girdle vessel ) that will regulate the quantity of vaginal discharge. ST-30, GB-26 will eliminate the dampness from the inferior burner. SP-10 regulates the blood, SP-9 and ST-36 eliminate the dampness. CV-3 eliminates the dampness from urination. From the differentiation of syndromes ( patterns ), the selection of points will be done. Medium level manipulation is used.

### <119> Female infertility

The causes can be systematic problems of sexual organs, overweight, mental problems, sexual inability or diabetes etc. Medical consultation is essential. In TCM, if no apparent causes are found, usually diagnose it as the coldness in uterus. Coldness can include various meanings like mal functions of sexual organs etc. But if the uterus' temperature is really low, the sperms are not able to survive. The overweight also can be a main cause that influence the hormone system and TCM explains that the phlegm ( overweight ) influences the CV channel and Chong mai ( penetrating vessel ) that are the main channels to regulate the menstruation and fertility. Deficiency of Qi, blood or inferior burner or stagnation of Qi or blood also can be the causes. The acupuncture can help the cases of infertility of functional problems or coldness in TCM.

The main points : TB-3 ( Zhong zhu ), GV-4 ( Ming men ), Liv-3 ( Tai chong ), SP-6 ( San yin jiao ), ST-36 ( Zu san li ), GV-20 ( Bai hui ), K-7 ( Fu liu ), Zi gong ( Ex ), BL-53 ( Bao huang ), BL-23 ( Shen shu )

The accompanying points : CV-12 ( Zhong wan ), Lu-7 ( Lie que ), SP-4 ( Gong sun ), BL-31 ( Shang liao ), K-6 ( Zhao hai ), LI-4 ( He gu ), ST-29 ( Gui lai ), SI-3 ( Hou xi ), BL-27 ( Xiao chang shu ), CV-6 ( Qi hai ), ST-28 ( Shui dao )

GV-4 is for the case of coldness in uterus. SP-4 activates the Chong mai ( penetrating vessel ), SI-3 activates the GV channel. Lu-7 activates the CV channel. BL-27, 23 and 31 can eliminate the dampness from the inferior burner and activate the circulation of uterus. TB-3 is for activating TB channel. Needles or moxibustion is used. Moxibustion is more effective.

### <120> Malpresentation or fetal malposition
It can be diagnosed after 30 weeks of pregnancy. Medical consultation is essential.

The main points : BL-67 ( Zhi yin )

BL-67 is the special point treat this problem. Needles or moxibustion can be used. Moxibustion is used for 30 minutes or medium level manipulation is used.

### <121> Mastitis
In TCM, problems on ST channel and Liv channel are the main causes of mastitis. Medical consultation is essential. The acute case with fever, redness, swollen and pain needs to be treated by cooling the heat, eliminating the pus and detoxification. In case of chronic and deficiency case, it is necessary to tonify. Liver qi stagnation or blood stagnation from the emotional stress can be the cause.

The main points : GB-21 ( Jian jing ), Liv-2 ( Xing jian ), CV-17 ( Shan zhong ), SI-1 ( Shao ze ), LI-11 ( Qu chi ), ST-37 ( Shang ju xu ), ST-40 ( Feng long ) : Bleeding method, ST-44 ( Nei ting ), LI-4 ( He gu ), ST-12 ( Que pen ), SI-11 ( Tian zong )

The accompanying points : LI-10 ( Shou san li ), GV-14 ( Da zhui ), ST-36 ( Zu san li ), BL-43 ( Gao huang ), SP-6 ( San yin jiao ), SP-18 ( Tian xi ), SP-9 ( Yin ling quan ), ST-15 ( Wu ye ), Liv-3 ( Tai chong )

Cooling the heat from the ST and Liv channel are used. In case of acute and heat are apparent, strong manipulation is used. In case of liver Qi stagnation from emotional stress is apparent, use more points to eliminate the Liver Qi stagnation.

### <122> Menopause disorder

In TCM the main causes are deficiency of Yin, Yang, or Qi stagnation etc. Medical consultation is essential. But the common symptoms usually show the Yin deficiency cases like night sweat, facial flush, heat on face, irritability etc. The main treatment principle is regulating the CV channel and Chong mai ( penetrating vessel ) and nourishing the body.

The main points : Liv-3 ( Tai chong ), Ht-6 ( Yin xi ), BL-23 ( Shen shu ), SP-4 ( Gong sun ), K-7 ( Fu liu ), LI-4 ( He gu ), SP-10 ( Xue hai ), K-6 ( Zhao hai ), SP-6 ( San yin jiao ), PC-6 ( Nei guan ), ST-44 ( Nei ting ), BL-17 ( Ge shu )

The accompanying points : BL-31 ( Shang liao ), Ht-7 ( Shen men ), BL-12 ( Feng men ), Lu-10 ( Yu ji ), LI-11 ( Qu chi ), Lu-5 ( Chi ze ) : bloodletting technique for heat, BL-15 ( Xin shu ), BL-63 ( Jin men ), CV-6 ( Qi hai ), GV-12 ( Shen zhu ), BL-18 ( Gan shu ), GV-14 ( Ming men ) for cold syndrome, An mian ( Ex ) for insomnia.

SP-4 activates the Chong mai ( penetrating vessel ). Lu-10 clears the heat from the superior burner. ST-44 clears the facial heat. Ht-6 is the Xi cleft point of heart channel and it stops night sweating. Ht-7 and PC-6 calms the mind. K-6 nourish the Kidneys. Strong manipulation is used for eliminating points and soft manipulation is used for nourishing points.

### <123> Menstrual irregularity

The blood color, quantity or property of blood or menstruation cycle are not normal. Medical consultation is essential. In TCM, this symptom is considered as irregular function of CV channel, Chong mai ( penetrating vessel ) or GV channel. Liv channel is related too in case emotional stress is involved. Deficiency of body also can cause menstrual irregularity.

The main points : SP-4 ( Gong sun ), Ht-7 ( Shen men ), Liv-3 ( Tai chong ), SP-10 ( Xue hai ), SP-6 ( San yin jiao ), SP-9 ( Yin ling quan ), CV-4 ( Guan yuan )
The accompanying points : BL-23 ( Shen shu ), Liv-2 ( Xing jian ), CV-3 ( Zhong ji ), PC-6 ( Nei guan ), LI-11 ( Qu chi ), Zi gong ( Ex ), ST-36 ( Zu san li ), GV-4 ( Ming men ), LI-4 ( He gu )

Medium level manipulation is used. SP-10 and Liv-2 are for blood stagnation or heat on Liv channel. ST-36 and SP-4 are for deficiency and SP-4 also activates Chong mai ( penetrating vessel ). PC-6 and Liv-3 are for irregular cycle. LI-11 can be used for heat. Zi gong is the special point for irregular menstruation and mal functions of ovaries. Soft manipulation can be used for CV-4 and GV-4 in case of deficiency case.

### <124> Menstrual pain

When the menstruation period is close, the patients suffer from abdominal pain, headache, palpitation or dizziness. Medical consultation is essential. There can be many different causes and syndrome patterns for menstrual pain but the main treatment principle is regulating CV channel, Chong mai ( penetrating vessel ) and relieving pain. The more points or different treatments can be added following the syndrome patterns.

The main points : Liv-3 ( Tai chong ), GB-31 ( Feng shi ), ST-34 ( Liang qiu ), SP-6 ( San yin jiao ), Zi gong ( Ex ), CV-4 ( Guan yuan )
The accompanying points : GB-20 ( Feng chi ), LI-4 ( He gu ), Shi qi zhui xia ( Ex ), ST-43 ( Xian gu ), PC-6 ( Nei guan ), CV-3 ( Zhong ji ), SP-4 ( Gong sun )

Zi gong is the special point to regulate the menstruation. Liv-3 and SP-6 regulate the menstruation. ST-34 relieves the abdominal pain. PC-6 calms the palpitation and SP-4 regulates Chong mai ( penetrating vessel ). Shi qi zhui xia is the local point of lumbar pain. ST-43 is for the migraine of menstruation. Strong manipulation is used. Treatment begins from 1 week before the menstruation period.

### <125> Oligomenorrhea, hypomenorrhea, Insufficient menstruation

This is a lack of quantity of blood in menstruation or excessively long cycle of menstruation. Medical consultation is essential. There are many causes like problems in ovaries, endocrine problems, sexual organs, and other internal diseases that influence the menstruation. In TCM, mainly the deficiency of blood, Yang, spleen Qi, phlegm, coldness or stagnation etc are responsible for this symptom.

The main points : SP-6 ( San yin jiao ), SP-10 ( Xue hai ), Liv-3 ( Tai chong ), BL-32 ( Ci liao ), LI-4 ( He gu ), BL-17 ( Ge shu ), BL-52 ( Zhi shi ), BL-23 ( Shen shu ), CV-4 ( Guan yuan ), BL-18 ( Gan shu ), K-7 ( Fu liu )

The accompanying points : ST-36 ( Zu san li ), GV-4 ( Ming men ), BL-27 ( Xiao chang shu ), GB-21 ( Jian jing ), Liv-9 ( Yin bao ), Zi gong ( Ex ), GV-20 ( Bai hui ), ST-27 ( Da ju ), K-6 ( Zhao hai )

In case of deficiency, CV-4, SP-6, BL-52, BL-23, SP-10, GV-4, GV-20 or K-6 can nourish or tonify the body. BL-32 regulates the menstruation and promote the circulation of blood at pelvis. GB-21 descends Qi downwards. And SP-10 is the special point for problems of blood. Zi gong regulate menstruation. BL-17 and BL-18 regulate the menstruation and nourish blood. Strong manipulation is used for the acute and excess pattern. Moxibustion can be used for cold or deficiency cases.

### <126> Painless or easy delivery

This method is used for the woman not to feel much pain at the time of delivery or for easy delivery. Medical consultation is essential to prepare for delivery. Generally the pain of delivery comes from the rhythmic movement of uterus at the time of delivery. The movement of uterus is inevitable but acupuncture can reduce the pain. The treatment is forbidden before 37the week of pregnancy.

The main points : BL-62 ( Shen mai ), BL-60 ( Kun lun ), Liv-3 ( Tai chong ), PC-8 ( Lao gong ), GB-34 ( Yang ling quan ), ST-36 ( Zu san li ), GB-21 ( Jian jing ), SP-6 ( San yin jiao ),

The accompanying points : LI-11 ( Qu chi ), SP-10 ( Xue hai ), PC-6 ( Nei guan ), K-8 ( Jiao xin ), PC-8 ( Lao gong ), Ht-7 ( Shen men ), LI-4 ( He gu )

This treatment shouldn't be done before 37th week of pregnancy because it can induce preterm birth. The treatment is done once a week from 38th week of pregnancy. SP-6 or K-8 and ST-36 promote the blood circulation of pelvis. GB-34 relieves the tension of muscle and tendons. PC-6 and Ht-7 calms the mind.

### <127> Postpartum hemorrhage

The main cause is when the uterine muscle does not contract enough to clamp the placental vessels shut. Medical consultation is essential. In TCM, the emergency points are used to avoid the danger and to stop bleeding.

The main points : Liv-3 ( Tai chong ), SP-6 ( San yin jiao ), BL-23 ( Shen shu ), GV-20 ( Bai hui ), Liv-1 ( Da dun ), CV-4 ( Guan yuan ), GB-34 ( Yang ling quan ), SP-1 ( Yin bai ), BL-17 ( Ge shu ), SP-10 ( Xue hai )

The accompanying points : BL-18 ( Gan shu ), K-9 ( Zhu bin ), SP-9 ( Yin ling quan ), BL-13 ( Fei shu ), K-7 ( Fu liu ), BL-32 ( Ci liao ), K-6 ( Zhao hai ), ST-36 ( Zu san li )

SP-1 and Liv-1 are Jing well points of emergency to stop bleeding. GV-20 directs qi upwards to stop bleeding. GB-34 regulates the uterine muscle. SP-10 and BL-17 regulate the blood. CV-4, K-6, BL-23, K-6 and K-7 nourish the body. Medium level manipulation is used.

### <128> Retroverted uterus

This is a common condition and it does not necessarily cause the serious problems but sometimes causes irregular menstruation, lumbar pain, infertility or endometriosis. Medical consultation is essential. The main causes are genetic problem, endometriosis, tumor or salpingitis etc. In TCM, this condition can be related with the problem of CV channel, Chong mai ( penetrating vessel ), GV channel or Liv channel. Depending on the symptoms that patient experience, the TCM syndromes can be different but usually regulating the above channels, vessel and local points that activate the circulation of blood in pelvis are the main idea of treatment.

The main points : CV-4 ( Guan yuan ), Liv-8 ( Qu quan ), SP-8 ( Di ji ), ST-36 ( Zu san li ), BL-23 ( Shen shu ), BL-33 ( Zhong liao ), ST-28 ( Shui dao ), Liv-3 ( Tai chong ), SP-6 ( San yin jiao )

The accompanying points : CV-12 ( Zhong wan ), TB-4 ( Yang chi ), Zi gong ( Ex ), BL-18 ( Gan shu ), SI-3 ( Hou xi ), K-8 ( Jiao xin ), K-14 ( Si man ), BL-32 ( Ci liao ), SP-10 ( Xue hai ), Lu-5 ( Chi ze ), BL-25 ( Da chang shu )

SP-6, Liv-3, CV-4, SP-10, SP-8 regulate the menstruation and relieve the pain of reverted uterus. The local points promote the circulation in the pelvis. Medium level manipulation is used. Zi gong is the extra acupoint for uterus.

### <129> Sexual insensitivity, frigidity

The causes are complicated because this condition is related with mental, emotional and physical conditions. If no apparent causes are detected from medical examination, it is worth trying acupuncture treatment. Medical consultation is essential. In TCM, Liv channel passes the sexual organ and treating and regulating this channel is the main idea. If there is mental stress, relieving the stress will be the main treatment idea. If the coldness is stagnated on Liv channel, the woman can feel pain with sexual activity and in that case, warming the channel is the main idea of treatment.

The main points : Liv-1 ( Da dun ), CV-3 ( Zhong ji ), PC-6 ( Nei guan ), CV-4 ( Guan yuan ), K-12 ( Da he ), Liv-3 ( Tai chong ), GV-4 ( Ming men ), K-7 ( Fu liu ), Liv-8 ( Qu quan )

The accompanying points : GV-12 ( Shen zhu ), TB-3 ( Zhong zhu ), BL-32 ( Ci liao ), PC-7 ( Da ling ), Ht-7 ( Shen men ), BL-23 ( Shen shu ), ST-36 ( Zu san li ), GV-20 ( Bai hui ), BL-17 ( Ge shu )

CV-4, BL-23 and GV-4 warms the inferior burner. Liv-3, PC-6, PC-7 and Ht-7 relieve the mental stress. Liv-1 activates the Liv channel. Local points near sexual organs are used to promote the circulation in the pelvis. Medium level manipulation is used.

### <130> Uterine cancer

There are many causes of uterine cancer, but the most commonly seen causes are obesity and emotional stress. Medical consultation is essential. All cancer patients must first go to the hospital to receive medical treatment and diagnosis from an oncologist. Acupuncture treatment can not replace medical treatment. Uterine cancer is related with sex hormones and menopausal state too. In TCM regulating the Qi and blood and eliminating the mass, detoxification method is used. Uterus is on the liver channel and Chong mai ( Penetrating vessel ). There are many cases of cold uterus. Regulating those channels is a essential part of management. Be careful not to needle on the tumor. You can refer to the section that discusses acupuncture and massage for cancer patients, which is located in the final part of this book.

Acupuncturists must adhere to acupuncture safety guidelines and comply with the acupuncture laws of their respective countries.

The main points : Liv-3 ( Tai chong ), Liv-8 ( Qu quan ), GB-26 ( Dai mai ), SP-6 ( San yin jiao ), TB-3 ( Zhong zhu ), ST-36 ( Zu san li )

The accompanying points : K-10 ( Yin gu ), SP-9 ( Yin ling quan ), K-11 ( Heng gu ), ST-28 ( Shui dao ), K-6 ( Zhao hai ), BL-32 ( Ci liao ), ST-27 ( Da ju ), SP-10 ( Xue hai )

For the cold syndromes, moxibustion is used on the acupoints of the lower abdomen like GB-26, ST-27, K-10, ST-28, K-11 rather than the needles. Generally, needles are not used on the local points of cancer mass or lower abdomen of uterine cancer. Liv-3 is the Yuan source point of the liver channel. Liv-3 and SP-6 liberate and regulate the liver channel and also SP-6 eliminates the dampness from the uterus. Liv-8 is the He sea point on the lower limbs. GB-26 eliminates the dampness on the lower burner. BL-32 activates and regulates the uterus. The accompanying points can be modified considering the situation of kidneys, liver and dampness. Soft or medium level manipulation is used.

### <131> Uterine fibroids ( Leiomyomas, Myomas )

Stagnation of Qi, blood and coldness in the uterus are the main causes of uterine fibroids. Medical consultation is essential. This is related with emotional stress, constitutional ( genetic ) condition and also originates from types of foods. The acupuncture treatment is to regulate the Qi and blood on the uterus region using channels.

The main points : Liv-3 ( Tai chong ), K-11 ( Heng gu ), ST-40 ( Feng long ), GV-8 ( Jin suo ), CV-4 ( Guan yuan ), SP-6 ( San yin jiao ), ST-25 ( Tian shu ), Ashi

The accompanying points : BL-25 ( Da chang shu ), SP-10 ( Xue hai ), CV-5 ( Shi men ), K-9 ( Zhu bin ), K-12 ( Da he ), K-13 ( Qi xue ), BL-32 ( Ci liao ), ST-36 ( Zu san li )

The treatment of regulating the Qi and blood using liver and kidneys channels and local points is used. Strong manipulation is used to eliminate the accumulation of fibroids. Moxibustion can be used too for the coldness syndrome. In case of deficiency condition, soft manipulation and tonifying points can be added.

### <132> Uterine prolapse

Uterine prolapse happens when the muscles and tissues of pelvis weaken. Medical consultation is essential. In TCM view the cause is original Qi deficiency and the Qi is sinking. The TCM main treatment idea is tonifying the original Qi and raise up the Qi.

The main points : CV-4 ( Guan yuan ), BL-32 ( Ci liao ), SP-6 ( San yin jiao ), GV-20 ( Bai hui ), ST-30 ( Qi chong ), Lu-7 ( Lie que ), Liv-3 ( Tai chong )
The accompanying points : Liv-8 ( Qu quan ), K-7 ( Fu liu ), GB-28 ( Wei dao ), Zi gong ( Ex ), K-3 ( Tai xi ), CV-6 ( Qi hai ), SP-6 ( Yin ling quan )

GV-20 tonifies the Qi and holds the Qi not to sink. ST-30 makes the Qi rise. CV-6 is to tonify the original Qi. Zi gong is the extra acupoint for uterus. The soft manipulation is used fot the tonifying acupoints and the strong manipulation is used for other points. The needle direction of GB-28 is to inner and lower area.

### <133> Vomiting with pregnancy ( Morning sickness )

The vomiting or nausea with pregnancy is a very common symptom but the main causes are not known. Medical consultation is essential. Probably the hormone changes can be related. In TCM view, the irregular upwards movement of the stomach Qi is the main cause.

The TCM treatment idea is to sink the stomach Qi and regulate the movement of Qi.

The main points : SP-4 ( Gong sun ), PC-6 ( Nei guan ), ST-36 ( Zu san li ), CV-12 ( Zhong wan )

The accompanying points : ST-44 ( Nei ting ), LI-10 ( Shou san li ), ST-40 ( Feng long )

CV-12 is the front mu point of stomach and it regulates the movement of stomach Qi. PC-6 and SP-4 are a combination to regulate the stomach and to sink the stomach Qi. ST-36 also has the function to sink the stomach Qi. ST-44 cools the stomach heat, ST-40 regulates the movement of Qi and eliminates the phlegm. Soft manipulation is used.

# | 15 |

# Headache

### <134> Headache – frontal area

There are many causes of headache but usually heat, coldness, deficiency, stagnation, phlegm etc. are related. Medical consultation is essential. Detail differentiation of syndromes and patterns are needed. Frontal headache is related with Yang ming channels like stomach and large intestine channels. The main idea of treatment in TCM is to regulate the Qi and blood in Yang ming channel.

The main points : SP-4 ( Gong sun ) : after needle, let the patient move the head, GV-22 ( Xin hui ), ST-36 ( Zu san li ), Yin tang ( Ex ), LI-4 ( He gu ), ST-44 ( Nei ting ), GB-20 ( Feng chi )

The accompanying points : BL-2 ( Zan zhu ), GB-31 ( Feng shi ), GB-14 ( Yang bai ), Tai yang ( Ex ) : bloodletting technique is used.

The large intestine and stomach channels are used. LI-4 is the special point for headache. Yin tang and Tai yang are the extra acupoint in the frontal head to regulate the local Qi and blood and also eliminate the wind. GV-22, GB-20 and Tai yang eliminate the wind. Strong manipulation is used for excess cases.

### <135> Headache – general

There are many causes of headache but usually heat, coldness, deficiency, stagnation, phlegm etc. are related. Medical consultation is essential. Detail differentiation of syndromes and patterns are needed. The Yang channels that connect with head are used to treat the headache. The main idea of treatment is to eliminate the wind, regulate the Qi and blood.

The main points : LI-4 ( He gu ), GB-20 ( Feng chi ), Tai yang ( Ex ) : bloodletting technique is used, GV-20 ( Bai hui ), Liv-3 ( Tai chong ), GB-31 ( Feng shi ), Er jian ( Auricular acupuncture ) : bloodletting technique

The accompanying points : GB-20 ( Feng chi ), Yin tang ( Ex ), Lu-7 ( Lie que ), Si shen cong ( Ex ), Liv-2 ( Xing jian ), Lu-9 ( Tai yuan ) : for pulsating pain, SP-4 ( Gong sun )

LI-4 is the special point for headache. LI-4 and Liv-3 can be used together to open the orifices and regulate the movement of Qi in whole body. Yin tang and Tai yang are the extra acupoints for headache. They regulate the Qi and blood of the head area. GB-20 eliminates the wind from the head. Lu-7 is the luo connecting point of lung channel and is also a special point for chornic headache. Si shen cong is the extra point on the head to eliminate the headache. It also calms the mind and treats the anxiety.

### <136> Migraine

Migraine is a severe headache that is usually accompanied by throbbing pain or pulsing sensation, usually on the sides of head. It also includes many other physical symptoms and prodromes. Medical consultation is essential. In TCM view the fire pathogen is the main cause. The treatment idea is to calm the fire and wind and to regulate the movement of Qi.

The main points : Liv-3 ( Tai chong ), GB-20 ( Feng chi ), LI-11 ( Qu chi ), TB-5 ( Wai guan ), TB-20 ( Jiao sun ), GB-5 ( Xuan lu ),

GB-41 ( Zu lin qi ), GV-20 ( Bai hui ), Er jian ( Auricular acupuncture ) : bloodletting technique

The accompanying points : GB-34 ( Yang ling quan ), GB-40 ( Qiu xu ), Lu-9 ( Tai yuan ), BL-7 ( Tong tian ), Tai yang ( Ex ) : bloodletting technique is used, TB-4 ( Yang chi )

The main acupoints are to eliminate the wind from the head and regulate the liver and gall bladder channel where the wind originates from. Lu-9 is the hui meeting point of pulsation to treat the throbbing pain or pulsing sensation. Bloodletting technique on the Tai yang point is used to eliminate the wind and calm the pain. Strong manipulation is used to eliminate the pathogens. In case of severe pain, bloodletting technique on Tai yang is used.

### <137> Occipital headache

The occipital region is where Tai yang channels like BL or SI passes through. Regulating the BL and SI channels are the essential point. Medical consultation is essential. As the all headaches originate from wind, eliminating the wind pathogen is necessary.

The main points : BL-40 ( Wei zhong ) : bloodletting technique, BL-10 ( Tian zhu ), GB-20 ( Feng chi ), BL-60 ( Kun lun ), GB-19 ( Nao kong ), SI-3 ( Hou xi )

The accompanying points : GV-16 ( Feng fu ), GB-21 ( Jian jing ), LI-4 ( He gu ), BL-62 ( Shen mai ), GV-14 ( Da zhui )

SI-3 is the distant point of occipital headache, it opens the governing vessel ( Du Mai ) and also regulates the SI channel. SI-3 and BL-62 are a combination to eliminate the pain from the occipital region. Bleeding on BL-40 can move blood and eliminate the blood stagnation. BL channel passes the occipital region and bloodletting technique on BL channel will relieve the pain. BL-62 is also the distant point for occipital pain. BL-10, GB-19 and GV-14 are the local point to eliminate the pain. LI-4 is the special point for headache. GB-20 and GV-16 eliminate the wind. BL-60 is the distant point for occipital headache. Strong manipulation is used to eliminate the pathogens. In case of severe pain, bloodletting technique on the area near GV-14 is used.

### <138> Occipital neuralgia

Pinched occipital nerves or tightness of muscles are the main causes of occipital neuralgia. Medical consultation is essential. In TCM, the main treatment idea is to relieve the tension on the occipital region and eliminate the wind from the head. It focuses on treating the channels of SI, BL, GB and GV

The main points : BL-10 ( Tian zhu ), GB-21 ( Jian jing ), GB-20 ( Feng chi ), BL-11 ( Da zhu ), BL-62 ( Shen mai ), SI-4 ( Wan gu ), GV-12 ( Shen zhu )

The accompanying points : GB-19 ( Nao kong ), GV-20 ( Bai hui ), SI-3 ( Hou xi ), BL-63 ( Jin men ), GV-16 ( Feng fu ), BL-40 ( Wei zhong ) : bloodletting technique

SI-3 and BL-62 are the combination to eliminate the pain from the occipital region. BL-10, GB-20 and BL-11 regulate the local Qi and eliminate the wind from the head. GV-20 regulates the Qi in the head. GV-16 eliminates the wind. SI-4 is the distant point for the occipital region. Strong manipulation is used to eliminate the pathogens. Bloodletting technique can be used on the local area of pain. SI-3 should be needled before BL-62.

### <139> Vertex headache

The liver channel, Du mai ( governing vessel ) are the main channels that pass through the vertex region of the head. Medical consultation is essential. Pathogens in the liver channel or emotional stress are the main causes of this problem. The main treatment idea is to eliminate the wind from the head specially using liver channel and Du mai.

The main points : GV-20 ( Bai hui ), GB-21 ( Jian jing ), Si shen cong ( Ex ), LI-4 ( He gu ), Liv-3 ( Tai chong ), Liv-1 ( Da dun ) : blood-letting technique

The accompanying points : PC-6 ( Nei guan ), GB-43 ( Xia xi ), Liv-2 ( Xing jian ), GV-22 ( Xin hui ), BL-7 ( Tong tian ), K-1 ( Yong quan )

Liv-3 and PC-6 regulate the liver Qi and relieve the mental stress. GV-20 and GV-22 eliminate the wind from the head. LI-4 is the special point for headache. K-1 is the distant point for the top of the head. BL-7 is the local acupoint and Si shen cong is the extra acupoint that treats the headache and anxiety. Strong manipulation is used to eliminate the pathogens. In case of severe pain, moxibustion on GV-20 and Si shen cong can be used.

# | 16 |

# Heart

**<140> Angina pectoris**

The main causes are hardening of the artery and it makes the heart muscle stressed. Medical consultation is essential. In TCM view, the stagnation of blood, phlegm, Qi are the main causes. Usually the fatty foods, lack of exercises, mental stress are closely related with this problem. The main treatment idea is to move blood and eliminate the blood stagnation on the chest.

The main points : Ht-7 ( Shen men ), SP-10 ( Xue hai ), Du yin ( Ex ) : bloodletting technique, Ht-9 ( Shao chong ), PC-4 ( Xi men ), SP-4 ( Gong sun ), PC-6 ( Nei guan ), PC-9 ( Zhong chong )

The accompanying points : CV-17 ( Shan zhong ), Ht-8 ( Shao fu ), bloodletting technique on the Jing well points at the emergency case., K-1 ( Yong quan ), Ht-6 ( Yin xi ), Liv-3 ( Tai chong )

SP-4 and PC-6 are the combination to treat the heart problem. They are the luo connecting point and relieve the qi and blood stagnation on the chest. They regulate the movement of qi and blood in heart too. Other points are about heart channels and to move Qi. K-1 has a good effect for emergency situation. Liv-3 activates the blood and Qi movement. Strong manipulation is used to remove the stagnation. Bloodletting technique on the Jing well points or under the second toe relieves the tightness on the heart. Du yin is the extra acupoint to move blood and stop pain. The location is on plantar side of second toe, on the center of the distal interphalangeal skin crease. The point under that second toe is called Huo bao. SP-4 should be needled before PC-6.

### <141> Endocarditis

The main cause is infection by bacteria or germs from the bloodstream. Medical consultation is essential. They stick to the heart valves or the damaged heart tissues. In TCM, there is no infection idea about this disease. The treatment idea in TCM is to regulate the Qi and blood of heart to relieve the pain and difficulty of breathing.

The main points : SP-4 ( Gong sun ), PC-6 ( Nei guan ), Ht-7 ( Shen men ), CV-17 ( Shan zhong ), BL-15 ( Xin shu ), Ht-1 ( Ji quan ), CV-14 ( Ju que )

The accompanying points : SI-11 ( Tian zong ), Ht-6 ( Yin xi ), PC-3 ( Qu ze ), BL-14 ( Jue yin shu ), PC-4 ( Xi men ), BL-15 ( Xin shu )

Medical treatment is necessary. Acupuncture is only for diminishing the pain temporarily. Strong manipulation is used to relieve the stagnation. The pericardium and heart channels are used to relieve the tension on the chest. SP-4 and PC-6 are the combination to relieve the pain on the chest. PC-4 is the Xi-cleft point of the pericardium channel to relieve the pain on the chest. Ht-1 is the Jing well point used for emergency case. BL-15 and 14 are the back shu point of heart and pericardium.

### <142> Heart pain

Heart pain can happen from various kinds of diseases. Medical consultation is essential. Here we talk about only the symptom, heart pain including chest pain. In TCM view, when the Qi and blood do not move freely, the pain happens. Also the dampness and phlegm can be related to this problem. The chest or heart area is the area of Qi and it is easily affected by emotional state. The main treatment idea is to open the chest and relieve the tension on the chest and heart. The treatment can be similar to angina pectoris because angina pectoris has the symptom of heart pain too. But if the cause of heart pain is known, that cause has to be treated first. Here we talk only about the treatment of the symptom, heart pain and not talk about the cause because there are too many causes.

The main points : CV-17 ( Shan zhong ), PC-6 ( Nei guan ), PC-4 ( Xi men ), SP-4 ( Gong sun ), Ht-3 ( Shao hai ), BL-14 ( Jue yin shu ), SP-10 ( Xue hai ), Liv-3 ( Tai chong )

The accompanying points : PC-9 ( Zhong chong ), GV-12 ( Shen zhu ), BL-15 ( Xin shu ), Ht-9 ( Shao chong ), SI-11 ( Tian zong ) on the left side, Du yin ( Ex ) : Bloodletting technique.

Relieving chest and heart tension is necessary. The local points on the chest, pericardium and heart channels are used. SP-4 and PC-6 are the combination to relieve the chest pain. BL-15 and BL-14 are the back shu points of heart and pericardium. The Jing well points and the Xi-cleft points are used to relieve the emergency pain. Du yin is the extra acupoint to move blood and stop pain. The location is on plantar side of second toe, on the center of the distal interphalangeal skin crease. Remove the needles right after strong manipulation is used. Bloodletting technique is used on Ht-9.

### <143> Palpitations

There are many causes and diseases that cause palpitations. Medical consultation is essential. The causes have to be treated first. In TCM view, heart fire, heart deficiency, blood deficiency or qi deficiency, phlegm etc. are the main pathology. These factors are closely related to emotion, foods and constitution etc. You can add more treatment for those pathological factors.

The main points : PC-8 ( Lao gong ), BL-15 ( Xin shu ), Ht-8 ( Shao fu ), Jing well points of hands, PC-6 ( Nei guan ), SP-4 ( Gong sun )

The accompanying points : PC-5 ( Jian shi ), CV-17 ( Shan zhong ), K-3 ( Tai xi ), Liv-3 ( Tai chong ), PC-4 ( Xi men ), Ht-7 ( Shen men ), CV-14 ( Ju que )

PC-6 is the luo connecting point of pericardium and it regulates the heart rate. Ht-8 cools the heart fire. CV-17 is the local point. CV-14 is the front mu point of heart. BL-15 is the back shu point of heart and PC-4 is the Xi-cleft point of pericardium. Ht-7 is the Yuan source point of heart. First, bloodletting technique on the Jing well points is used. Strong manipulation is used in case of excess syndrome.

### <144> Valvular heart disease

This disease happens when one or more heart valves do not properly close or open. Medical consultation is essential. The whooshing sound is heard through stethoscope. The patient can have chest pain, fatigue, abdominal swelling, short breathing or fatigue etc. In TCM view this can be interpreted in many syndromes and TCM diseases like palpitation, chest pain, fatigue etc. But if we know the heart valve has the problem through medical examination, we can choose the acupoint more for the heart issue. As such, medical examination can help TCM treatment in some way.

The main points : PC-3 ( Qu ze ), K-6 ( Zhao hai ), Liv-3 ( Tai chong ), GV-11 ( Shen dao ), Ht-7 ( Shen men ), PC-6 ( Nei guan ), BL-15 ( Xin shu )

The accompanying points : GB-34 ( Yang ling quan ), SP-10 ( Xue hai ), TB-15 ( Tian liao ), CV-17 ( Shan zhong ), SI-11 ( Tian zong ), BL-14 ( Jue yin shu ), GV-9 ( Zhi yang ), PC-4 ( Xi men )

BL-15 and BL-14 are the back shu points of heart and pericardium. GV-11, TB-15 and CV-17 are the local points to regulate the Qi and blood in the heart. Ht-7 is the Yuan source point of heart. PC-6 is the luo connecting point for pericardium. GV-9 is to open the chest. GB-34 is the hui meeting point of tendon because valve is a family of muscle and tendon. PC-4 is the Xi-cleft point of pericardium. Medical treatment is necessary. Acupuncture is only for diminishing the symptoms. Needles are used for the acute cases and moxibustion is used for chronic cases.

# | 17 |

# Internal problems

### <145> Abdominal pain

There are many causes of abdominal pain. Medical consultation is essential. The upper abdomen is related with stomach and the lower abdomen is more about liver, kidneys or intestine. The detailed diagnosis is necessary to differentiate the causes. If you know the causes or origin diseases, those causes or origin diseases have to be treated first. In TCM view, the methods of relieving abdominal tension, activating the movement of digestive system, eliminating coldness or heat are used.

The main points : ST-43 ( Xian gu ), BL-60 ( Kun lun ), LI-11 ( Qu chi ), ST-44 ( Nei ting ), Liv-2 ( Xing jian ), ST-36 ( Zu san li ), SP-1 ( Yin bai ), PC-6 ( Nei guan )

The accompanying points :

For upper abdomen pain : CV-12 ( Zhong wan ), ST-40 ( Feng long ), Lu-10 ( Yu ji ), ST-34 ( Liang qiu ), SP-4 ( Gong sun )

For lower abdomen pain : ST-37 ( Shang ju xu ), CV-4 ( Guan yuan ), CV-6 ( Qi hai ), SI-6 ( Yang lao ), SP-6 ( San yin jiao ), ST-25 ( Tian shu )

ST-44 and liv-2 eliminate the heat and excessive tension of abdomen. SP-1 is the Jing well point for the emergency pain. ST-34 is the Xi-cleft point of stomach to relieve the stomach pain. SP-4 and PC-6 regulate the stomach. SP-6 regulates the lower abdomen. ST-37 is the lower he sea point of large intestine. SI-6 is the Xi-cleft point of small intestine. First, strong manipulation on feet is used. In severe case, moxibustion is used on CV-6 for lower abdominal pain and CV-12 for upper abdominal pain.

### <146> Accumulation in heart ( Xin ji ) – five accumulation ( Wu ji ) (1)

This is a TCM disease name. Usually there are five kinds of accumulation in Zang organs. Accumulation in heart is called Fu liang. This disease is similar to a cyst or mass on the local area. Accumulation in heart has the mass from belly button to the area around CV14. If not treated properly, the patient will feel tightness on the chest. In TCM, the accumulation in the Zang organ happens with many causes. Emotional instability will hurt the organs and make them deficient. Those deficient organs will get the pathogens and a mass will grow. This is the origin of accumulation in Zang organs. The treatment idea of accumulation in heart is to eliminate the stagnation of Qi and blood, soften the mass.

The main points : SP-10 ( Xue hai ), CV-14 ( Ju que ), PC-6 ( Nei guan ), CV-17 ( Shan zhong ), Ht-7 ( Shen men ), BL-17 ( Ge shu )

The accompanying points : Liv-2 ( Xing jian ), BL-15 ( Xin shu ), CV-13 ( Shang wan ), SP-6 ( San yin jiao ), PC-7 ( Da ling ), Liv-3 ( Tai chong )

The local points, the heart and pericardium channels are used to eliminate the stagnation on the heart and pericardium. BL-17 is the hui meeting point of blood to eliminate the stagnation of blood. CV-14 is the front mu point of heart. Strong manipulation is used. Moxibustion is used on CV-13.

## <147> Accumulation in kidneys ( Shen ji ) – five accumulation ( Wu ji ) (2)

This is a TCM disease name. Usually there are five kinds of accumulation in Zang organs. Accumulation in kidneys is called Pen tun. This disease is similar to a cyst or mass on the local area. Accumulation in kidneys has the mass from lower abdomen to the area around CV14. Something fast is going up and down and it is like a pig. That is the origin of the disease name, Ben tun ( running pig ). If not treated properly, the patient will feel shortness of breath, weak bones and fatigue. In TCM, the accumulation in the Zang organ happens with many causes. Emotional instability will hurt the organs and make them deficient. Those deficient organs will get the pathogens and a mass will grow. This is the origin of accumulation in Zang organs. The treatment idea of accumulation in kidneys is to eliminate the stagnation of Qi and blood, soften the mass and strengthen the kidneys and bones.

The main points : GB-25 ( Jing men ), BL-23 ( Shen shu ), K-3 ( Tai xi ), Liv-13 ( Zhang men ), CV-4 ( Guan yuan ), SP-4 ( Gong sun )

The accompanying points : CV-12 ( Zhong wan ), SP-6 ( San yin jiao ), BL-64 ( Jing gu ), K-1 ( Yong quan ), CV-6 ( Qi hai ), CV-3 ( Zhong ji ), K-7 ( Fu liu )

BL-23 is the back shu point of kidneys. K-1 is the Jing well point to nourish the kidneys and relieve the pain. GB-25 is the front mu point of kidneys. K-3 is the Yuan source point of kidneys. BL-64 is the Yuan source point of urinary bladder. CV-3 activates the kidneys and urination. Liv-13 is the hui meeting point of Zang organ. CV-4 strengthens the kidneys and Qi. Strong manipulation is used. Moxibustion is used on CV-4.

## <148> Accumulation in liver ( Gan ji ) – five accumulation ( Wu ji ) (3)

This is a TCM disease name. Usually there are five kinds of accumulation in Zang organs. Accumulation in liver is called Fei qi. This disease is similar to a cyst or mass on the local area. Accumulation in liver has the mass from at the left side under the ribs. It is like a form of reverted liquor cup. If not treated properly, the patient will have hiccups, rib pains or alternating fever and cold. In TCM, the accumulation in the Zang organ happens with many causes. Emotional instability will hurt the organs and make them deficient. Those deficient organs will get the pathogens and a mass will grow. This is the origin of accumulation in Zang organs. The treatment idea of accumulation in liver is to eliminate the stagnation of Qi and blood, soften the mass on the local area.

The main points : PC-6 ( Nei guan ), Liv-13 ( Zhang men ), TB-6 ( Zhi gou ), BL-17 ( Ge shu ), Liv-3 ( Tai chong ), Liv-14 ( Qi men )

The accompanying points : GB-31 ( Feng shi ), Liv-2 ( Xing jian ), ST-36 ( Zu san li ), GB-41 ( Zu lin qi ), GV-14 ( Da zhui ), GB-34 ( Yang ling quan )

Liv-13 is the hui meeting point of Zang organs. Liv-14 is the front mu point of liver. BL-17 moves blood to eliminate the mass. Liv-3 is the Yuan source point of liver and it moves Qi and blood. GV-14 opens the Yang channels and clears the heat. ST-36 regulates the movement of Qi. GB-34 eliminates the dampness and nourishes the tendons. TB-6 regulates the movement of Qi on three burners and also activates the kidneys. Strong manipulation is used. Moxibustion is used on Liv-13.

### <149> Accumulation in lungs ( Fei ji ) – Wu ji, five accumulation (4)

This is a TCM disease name. Usually there are five kinds of accumulation in Zang organs. Accumulation in lung is called Xi pen. This disease is similar to a cyst or mass on the local area. Accumulation in lung has the mass at the right side under the ribs and it is like the reverted liquor cup. If not treated properly, the patient will feel alternating fever and coldness, shortness of breath, coughing and lung inflammation. In TCM, the accumulation in the Zang organ happens with many causes. Emotional instability will hurt the organs and make them deficient. Those deficient organs will get the pathogens and a mass will grow. This is the origin of accumulation in Zang organs. The treatment idea of accumulation in lung is to eliminate the stagnation of Qi and blood, soften the mass on the lung.

The main points : Lu-9 ( Tai yuan ), BL-13 ( Fei shu ), Lu-10 ( Yu ji ), Liv-13 ( Zhang men ), CV-14 ( Ju que ), Lu-8 ( Jing qu ), Liv-3 ( Tai chong )

The accompanying points : ST-40 ( Feng long ), CV-12 ( Zhong wan ), TB-6 ( Zhi gou ), LI-4 ( He gu ), Lu-1 ( Zhong fu ), Liv-14 ( Qi men ), PC-6 ( Nei guan ), ST-36 ( Zu san li )

Most of special points of lung channels are used. BL-13 is the back shu point of lung. Lu-8 regulates the movement of lung and treats coughing. Lu-9 is the Yuan source point of lung. TB-6 regulates the movement of breath. CV-14 is the front mu point of heart and it regulates the movement of breath. Liv-14 regulates the liver Qi and makes the breathing and movement of lung smoother. ST-40 eliminates the phlegm. PC-6 regulates the chest and lung. Liv-13 is the hui meeting point of Zang organ. Strong manipulation is used. Moxibustion is used on Liv-13.

### <150> Accumulation in spleen ( Pi ji ) – five accumulation ( Wu ji ) (5)

This is a TCM disease name. Usually there are five kinds of accumulation in Zang organs. Accumulation in spleen is called Pi qi. This disease is similar to a cyst or mass on the local area. Accumulation in spleen has the mass at the area around CV-12 and the mass can be located a little at the right side of it. It is like a reverted liquor cup or plate. If not treated properly, the patient can not move four limbs properly or can have jaundice and becomes skinny. In TCM, accumulation in the Zang organ happens with many causes. Emotional instability will hurt the organs and make them deficient. Those deficient organs will get the pathogens and a mass will grow. This is the origin of accumulation in Zang organs. The treatment idea of accumulation in spleen is to eliminate the stagnation of Qi and blood, soften the mass on the spleen.

The main points : SP-9 ( Yin ling quan ), SP-4 ( Gong sun ), PC-6 ( Nei guan ), CV-13 ( Shang wan ), Liv-3 ( Tai chong ), Pi gen ( Ex ), SP-6 ( San yin jiao )
The accompanying points : ST-36 ( Zu san li ), ST-40 ( Feng long ), BL-20 ( Pi shu ), SP-1 ( Yin bai ), ST-44 ( Nei ting ), Liv-2 ( Xing jian ), CV-12 ( Zhong wan )

SP-4 is the luo connecting point of spleen and it eliminates the dampness and also nourishes the blood and Yin. SP-4 and PC-6 are the combination to regulate the chest and stomach area. Pi gen is the extra acupoint to eliminate the mass or cyst. BL-20 is the back shu point of spleen. SP-1 is the Jing well point of spleen channel and removes the heat and relieves the pain on the spleen channel. CV-12 is the front mu point of stomach and also hui meeting point of Fu organs to regulate the spleen and stomach Qi. ST-44 eliminates the heat on the spleen. ST-36 regulates the movement of Qi in spleen and stomach. Strong manipulation is used. Moxibustion is used on CV-12.

### <151> Addison's disease, Chronic adrenal insufficiency
This disease happens because the adrenal glands generate too little cortisol or aldosterone. This is life threatening and the patient needs to take the hormone to replace those that are missing. Medical consultation is essential. The patient will experience severe fatigue, weight loss, loss of appetite, dehydration, low blood pressure or low blood sugar etc. In TCM view this is deficiency of Qi, collapse of Qi or

deficiency of kidneys Qi. The main treatment idea it is to strengthen the kidneys and Qi.

The main points : BL-20 ( Pi shu ), BL-32 ( Ci liao ), K-7 ( Fu liu ), GV-4 ( Ming men ), CV-4 ( Guan yuan ), BL-23 ( Shen shu ), GV-12 ( Shen zhu ), BL-52 ( Zhi shi ), ST-36 ( Zu san li )

The accompanying points : GV-20 ( Bai hui ), BL-17 ( Ge shu ), SP-8 ( Di ji ), K-3 ( Tai xi ), CV-12 ( Zhong wan ), K-16 ( Huang shu ), BL-10 ( Tian zhu )

GV-12 activates the Yang qi. BL-17 nourishes blood and also activates the liver. BL-20 activates spleen. BL-23 strengthens the kidneys to generate the hormones. BL-52 nourishes kidneys essence and strengthens the kidneys. BL-32 activates kidneys. CV-6 strengthens Qi. K-16 strengthens kidneys. ST-36 strengthens Qi. K-3 is the Yuan source point of kidneys to nourish kidneys. SP-8 moves blood also nourishes spleen to help tonify Qi and nourish blood. Medium level manipulation is used. Needles are used on acute case and moxibustion is used on chronic case.

### <152> Anemia

The western medical diagnosis of anemia and TCM anemia ( deficiency of blood ) are not exactly same. Medical consultation is essential. If the symptoms like weak memory, insomnia, pale color of face and lips, dizziness, thin pulse etc. are diagnosed as deficiency of blood in TCM. Western medical anemia is about a lack of iron or irregularity of blood cells etc. The blood is produced from bone marrow and vitamin B12 is joining on the process. Also the blood production stimulants that are generated from kidneys are also an important factor to produce blood. Here the anemia can include the both meanings. In TCM view, the treatment idea is to strengthen the spleen and kidneys to produce more blood and move blood.

The main points : SP-10 ( Xue hai ), CV-6 ( Qi hai ), BL-20 ( Pi shu ), CV-4 ( Guan yuan ), ST-36 ( Zu san li ), BL-23 ( Shen shu ), BL-17 ( Ge shu ), SP-6 ( San yin jiao ), GV-20 ( Bai hui )

The accompanying points : BL-18 ( Gan shu ), GV-4 ( Ming men ), BL-23 ( Shen shu ), BL-12 ( Feng men ), CV-5 ( Shi men ), CV-12 ( Zhong wan ), LI-11 ( Qu chi ), SP-4 ( Gong sun ), SI-3 ( Hou xi )

CV-4, CV-5 or CV-6 strengthens Qi, liver or kidneys to tonify Qi and blood. ST-36 strengthens Qi. BL-23 activates kidneys to generate Qi. GV-4 activates kidneys Yang. BL-20 strengthens spleen. BL-12 is the point to eliminate the wind and also to strengthen lung to activate kidneys. LI-11 clears the body heat that can be a origin of anemia and also activates large intestine. BL-17 eliminates the wind of deficiency of blood from lung and also because blood is generated in lung in TCM view. Moxibustion is more effective than needles.

### <153> Arteriosclerosis

When the blood vessels from the heart are hardened and become thick, the blood flow from heart is restricted. Medical consultation is essential. When the blood vessels are blocked by plaque, it is called Atherosclerosis and it is a special type of arteriosclerosis. The patients can experience chest pain, numb limbs or dizziness etc. In TCM view, this is the deficiency of heart, deficiency of blood or blood stagnation. The main treatment idea is to activate the blood, nourish the heart, move blood and eliminate the blood stagnation to activate the flow.

The main points : LI-11 ( Qu chi ), SP-10 ( Xue hai ), GV-20 ( Bai hui ), ST-36 ( Zu san li ), LI-10 ( Shou san li ), PC-6 ( Nei guan ), SP-4 ( Gong sun ), BL-15 ( Xin shu ), BL-14 ( Jue yin shu )

The accompanying points : GB-39 ( Xuan zhong ), SP-6 ( San yin jiao ), GB-31 ( Feng shi ), BL-17 ( Ge shu ), GB-7 ( Qu bin ), GB-21 ( Jian jing ), GB-20 ( Feng chi ), CV-12 ( Zhong wan ), BL-18 ( Gan shu )

ST-36 and GB-39 strengthen the heart and activate the blood flow. LI-10 strengthens the spleen. LI-11 harmonizes the Qi. PC-6 regulates the movement of heart. SP-6 nourishes blood and Yin. GV-20 holds the Qi. GB-20 eliminates the wind from the brain. GB-31 eliminates the wind to prevent ACV. GB-21 regulates the movement of Qi. Moxibustion is used on ST-36 and GB-39. Needles are used on other points with medium level manipulation.

### <154> Ascites

Ascites easily happens with cirrhosis, kidneys conditions or malnutrition. Medical consultation is essential. The patients usually experience discomfort on the abdomen, nausea, vomit or shortness of breath. In TCM view, the causes are complex. There are liver and spleen issues, dampness and stagnation of qi or blood, deficiency of Yang of kidneys etc. Most of all, the first thing to do in acupuncture is to eliminate the dampness and stagnation of water. And following the syndromes or patterns, you can add more treatments. Here we focus on eliminating the water stagnation.

The main points : CV-9 ( Shui fen ), SP-9 ( Yin ling quan ), ST-28 ( Shui dao ), ST-30 ( Qi chong ), CV-7 ( Yin jiao ), K-7 ( Fu liu ), ST-40 ( Feng long )

The accompanying points : K-10 ( Yin gu ), K-2 ( Ran gu ), BL-13 ( Xin shu ), K-3 ( Tai xi ), BL-23 ( Shen shu ), BL-39 ( Wei yang ), Liv-2 ( Xing jian ), BL-20 ( Pi shu ), BL-18 ( Gan shu )

CV-9 activates the water movement and eliminates the liquid stagnation from the body. ST-30 activates the Yang Ming Qi to move Qi from the lower burner to eliminate the liquid stagnation. BL-39 promotes urination to eliminate the water stagnation. K-2 eliminates the heat from the urinary tract or kidneys. CV-7 and ST-28 promotes the movement of water. BL-23 is the back shu point of kidneys. BL-13 and K-3 are used to activate the heart and kidneys to promote the functions. K-10 strengthens the kidneys. Soft manipulation is used. Moxibustion on ST-30, CV-7 or K-10 are used.

### <155> Bad breath ( halitosis )

The bad breath can happen with some dental conditions or stomach problems. Medical consultation is essential. Here we focus only on stomach problems because dental conditions can be improved with proper dental hygiene. In TCM view, usually stomach heat is the main cause. Absorption of too much spicy food, stimulating foods like caffeine or deficiency of stomach can accumulate foods and also can make bad breath. The main treatment idea is to clear the stomach heat and to regulate the movement of stomach to make it function normally.

The main points : ST-42 ( Chong yang ), LI-11 ( Qu chi ), ST-36 ( Zu san li ), CV-12 ( Zhong wan ), ST-44 ( Nei ting ), SP-4 ( Gong sun ), PC-6 ( Nei guan )

The accompanying points : LI-10 ( Shou san li ), BL-21 ( Wei shu ), CV-10 ( Xia wan ), CV-13 ( Shang wan ), SP-6 ( San yin jiao )

ST-44 clears the stomach heat. ST-36 regulates the movement of stomach. ST-42 strengthens stomach. CV-12 is the hui meeting point of fu organs and front mu point of stomach. BL-21 is the back shu point of stomach. CV-13 and CV-10 are the local points to regulate the stomach. SP-4 is the luo connecting points of spleen channel to treat the chronic case of stomach. LI-10 strengthens spleen and activates the stomach. Strong manipulation is used for the excess case and soft manipulation is used for those strengthening points.

### <156> Beriberi, thiamine deficiency

Beriberi is a kind of disease that the patient is in lack of vitamin B1. Medical consultation is essential. The symptoms are usually fatigue, weight loss, difficulty in digesting the carbohydrates, weak memory, abdominal discomfort etc. The treatment is to take the vitamin B1 and other nutrients. But with acupuncture treatment, the recovery can be faster. In TCM view, the main treatment idea is to strengthen limbs, Qi and blood to tonify the body.

The main points : ST-35 ( Du bi ), SP-10 ( Xue hai ), ST-37 ( Shang ju xu ), BL-20 ( Pi shu ), GB-39 ( Xuan zhong ), ST-36 ( Zu san li ), ST-39 ( Xia ju xu ), CV-4 ( Guan yuan )

The accompanying points : CV-14 ( Ju que ), GV-20 ( Bai hui ), CV-12 ( Zhong wan ), BL-25 ( Da chang shu ), BL-15 ( Xin shu ), GB-31 ( Feng shi ), ST-32 ( Fu tu ), GV-12 ( Shen zhu ), Nei xi yan ( Ex )

GB-31 eliminates the wind and strengthens the lower limb. ST-32, Nei xi yan, ST-36 and ST-35 strengthens the lower limbs. ST-37, ST-39 and GB-39 strengthen the lower limbs and activities Qi. The accompanying points are to activate the digestion system to produce more Qi and blood. BL-15 activates heart to nourish blood. GV-12 strengthens the bone and Yang qi. Needles are used with medium level manipulation on acute case. Moxibustion is used on chronic case.

### <157> Carsickness, seasickness or airsickness ( motion sickness )

The symptoms are nausea, vomit, cold sweat, headache, dizziness, tiredness or loss of appetite. In TCM view, this problem is based on heat and dampness of middle burner that excites the stomach and blocks the regular movement of Qi, deficiency of middle burner that causes irregular movement of Qi. The main treatment idea is to regulate the movement of Qi, activate the middle burner and clear the heat of the spleen and stomach.

The main points : PC-6 ( Nei guan ), SP-4 ( Gong sun ), CV-12 ( Zhong wan ), ST-44 ( Nei ting ), ST-36 ( Zu san li ), An mian ( Ex )

The accompanying points : ST-25 ( Tian shu ), TB-4 ( Yang chi ), BL-23 ( Shen shu ), SP-6 ( San yin jiao ), BL-18 ( Gan shu ), GV-22 ( Xin hui )

TB-4 regulates the movement of Qi upwards and downwards. SP-4 and PC-6 regulate the movement of Qi on middle burner to calm the motion sickness. ST-44 clears the stomach heat and calms the excitation of stomach. ST-25 regulates the Qi of digestion system. GV-22 calms the mind. BL-18 nourishes liver. BL-23 strengthens the kidneys and Qi. CV-12 regulates the fu organs. ST-36 eliminates the dampness and regulates the movement of Qi and strengthens the spleen and stomach. An mian is the extra acupoint to treat the insomnia but it also calms the mind. SP-6 nourishes the spleen and eliminates the dampness. Medium level manipulation is used.

### <158> Chest pain

Chest pain can include various cases like heart problem, lung problem or even emotional depression can show chest pain and tightness. Here we focus on the treatment of pain itself. Medical consultation is essential. In TCM view, the main treatment idea is to regulate the Qi and blood on the local area and relieve the pain. If any other syndromes or diseases of cause are known, the treatment has to be focused on those causes or additional treatment has to be added.

The main points : Liv-3 ( Tai chong ), PC-6 ( Nei guan ), SP-21 ( Da bao ), ST-18 ( Ru gen ), BL-15 ( Xin shu ), SP-4 ( Gong sun ), Liv-14 ( Qi men ), BL-17 ( Ge shu )

The accompanying points : ST-40 ( Feng long ), GB-34 ( Yang ling quan ), SI-11 ( Tian zong ), TB-6 ( Zhi gou ), Lu-7 ( Lie que ), K-6 ( Zhao hai )

SP-4 and PC-6 are the combination that regulates the movement of Qi and blood at the chest area to relieve the pain. SI-11 eliminates the stagnation at the local area. BL-15 and BL-17 regulates the blood.

SP-21 is the grand luo connecting point that relieves the pain on the chest. Lu-7 and K-6 are the combination to relieve the pain from lung. ST-18, Liv-14 and GB-34 regulate the liver Qi and eliminate the Qi stagnation of liver and local area. Strong manipulation is used to eliminate the Qi stagnation. Needle SP-4 before PC-6. Needle Lu-7 before K-6.

### <159> Diabetes mellitus, syndrome of consumptive thirst

Medical consultation is essential. Consumptive thirst is a TCM syndrome name that seems to be similar to diabetes mellitus but they are not exactly same. The diabetes mellitus has various syndromes or patterns and you need to analyze the patterns in detail to treat it. Syndrome of consumptive thirst is a kind of syndrome pattern that usually shows thirst, excessive eating or frequent urination. But diabetes mellitus does not always show the symptoms of consumptive thirst. Treatment of general diabetes mellitus is complicated because there are many complicated syndrome patterns. So, here we focus on the diabetes mellitus that shows the symptoms of consumptive thirst. But you still can use the main points in this prescription for the general diabetes mellitus too because it nourishes the body and can be used for most of diabetes mellitus cases.

The main points : BL-23 ( Shen shu ), Lu-9 ( Tai yuan ), ST-36 ( Zu san li ), BL-20 ( Pi shu ), Cui shu ( Ex ), BL-13 ( Fei shu ), K-3 ( Tai xi ), SP-6 ( San yin jiao )

The accompanying points :

For excessive urine : K-5 ( Shui quan ), K-7 ( Fu liu ), GV-20 ( Bai hui ), CV-4 ( Guan yuan )

For excessive appetite and fast digestion : LI-11 ( Qu chi ), BL-21 ( Wei shu ), ST-44 ( Nei ting ), CV-12 ( Zhong wan ), Pi re ( Ex )

For dry mouth : K-2 ( Ran gu ), Lu-10 ( Yu ji ), Lu-11 ( Shao shang ), K-6 ( Zhao hai )

Cui shu is the extra acupoints on the middle back, 1.5 cun lateral to the lower border of the spinous process of the eighth thoracic vertebra (T8). Cui shu is at the height of pancreas and it activates the function of pancreas. BL-13, BL-20 and BL-23 nourish the lung, spleen and kidneys. ST-36 increases the Qi and K-3 nourishes the essence of kidneys. The accompanying points for upper burner, middle burner and lower burner are to clear the heat on those areas and nourish Yin to relieve the consumptive symptoms. Soft manipulation is used on the back shu points. Pi re is the extra acupoint to treat problems of spleen and pancreas like inflammation of pancreas, heat, difficulty in digestion or enlarged spleen. It is located on the back, between the spinous processes of the 6th and 7th thoracic vertebrae, 0.5 cun apart on both sides, for a total of 2 acupuncture points. Medium level manipulations are used on other points.

### <160> Drowning

Drowning is an emergency situation. Firstly, emergency medical treatment has to be done. Medical consultation is essential. Acupuncture can be applied for those cases when recovery is delayed after the emergency medical treatment is done. The main treatment idea is to open the orifice to make the consciousness come back and activate the lung and Qi.

The main points : PC-6 ( Nei guan ), Lu-9 ( Tai yuan ), GV-25 ( Su liao ), K-1 ( Yong quan )

The accompanying points : GV-26 ( Shui gou ), ST-36 ( Zu san li ), SI-3 ( Hou xi ), CV-1 ( Hui yin ) : follow the safety guide of acupuncture

Other method : Moxibustion on the CV-12 ( Zhong wan ) or CV-8 ( Shen que )

GV-25, K-1 and PC-6 open the orifices and help the consciousness come back. Lu-9, SI-3 and ST-36 activate and regulate the Qi. At first, Emergency treatment is necessary. Strong manipulation is used.

## <161> Edema

There are many causes of edema like problems of heart, kidneys or liver. Medical consultation is essential. If the pathological organ is known, the treatment has to be focused on that organ. Here we focus on the eliminating the stagnation of water to treat the edema itself. The main treatment idea is to activate liver, kidneys, heart and promote urination. Strengthening Qi and Yang has special meaning to remove the water.

The main points : Liv-13 ( Zhang men ), ST-40 ( Feng long ), SP-9 ( Yin ling quan ), CV-9 ( Shui fen ), CV-6 ( Qi hai ), Liv-3 ( Tai chong ), K-3 ( Tai xi ), BL-18 ( Gan shu ), BL-40 ( Wei zhong ), BL-23 ( Shen shu )

The accompanying points :

For heart problem –BL-15 ( Xin shu ), Ht-7 ( Shen men ), BL-17 ( Ge shu ), PC-4 ( Xi men )

For kidneys problem – BL-52 ( Zhi shi ), K-7 ( Fu liu ), CV-4 ( Guan yuan ), K-1 ( Yong quan )

BL-18 is the back shu point of liver and it activates the liver. BL-23 is the back shu point of kidneys and it activates the kidneys. Liv-13 is the hui meeting point of Zang organ and is used for all kinds of Zang organ problems. CV-9 activates the Yang and promotes the urination. CV-6 strengthens the Qi. BL-40 promotes the urination. Liv-3 is the Yuan source point of liver and treats liver. K-3 is the Yuan source point of kidneys and treats kidneys. The accompanying points are specially for activating the functions of heart and kidneys in those cases. Strong manipulation is used to eliminate the pathogen but in case of fatigue and weakness, soft manipulation is used. In case of kidneys problem, moxibustion is used.

## <162> Electric shock

Electric shock is the emergency situation and the emergency medical treatment has to be do first. Medical consultation is essential. The acupuncture can be used for those cases when the recovery is delayed after the medical treatment. The main treatment idea is to open the orifices to awaken the consciousness, strengthen the Qi and regulate the Qi of heart to recover.

The main points : PC-6 ( Nei guan ), GV-23 ( Shui gou ), GV-25 ( Su liao ), K-1 ( Yong quan ), GV-20 ( Bai hui ), Yin tang ( Ex ), Xing fen ( Ex )

The accompanying points : CV-12 ( Zhong wan ), LI-4 ( He gu ), Ht-9 ( Shao chong ), ST-36 ( Zu san li )

Xing fen is the extra acupoint. Xing fen means excitation. Xing fen is located in the temporal part of the head, the posterior edge of the temporal bone mastoid and 0.5 cun above the depression under the mastoid, and 0.5 cun diagonally above the extra point of An mian. Xing fen point activates the heart beat and is used when the heart beat rate is too slow. GV-25 stimulates the heart and increases the blood pressure to recover from the shock. PC-6 regulates the heart movement. K-1 is used for the emergency shock cases. Ht-9 is the Jing well point to treat the emergency case. GV-20 activates the Qi to go upwards. Soft manipulation is used. Light moxibustion on ST-36 is used.

### <163> Feel cold

Feeling cold without any infection is not necessarily a disease but in TCM view, abnormal coldness on body is considered as pathological. Medical consultation is essential. The causes are various but here we focus on the deficiency of kidneys Yang and Qi case. The main treatment idea is to strengthen the Yang of kidneys and Qi to warm the body.

The main points : CV-12 ( Zhong wan ), GV-4 ( Ming men ), BL-23 ( Shen shu ), CV-8 ( Shen que ), ST-27 ( Da ju ), Ashi, CV-4 ( Guan yuan ), BL-20 ( Pi shu ), CV-6 ( Qi hai ), ST-36 ( Zu san li )

The accompanying points : K-10 ( Yin gu ), GV-3 ( Yao yang guan ), Liv-3 ( Tai chong ), BL-32 ( Ci liao ), SP-6 ( San yin jiao ), K-7 ( Fu liu ), K-3 ( Tai xi ), SP-10 ( Xue hai )

ST-36 strengthens the Qi. K-3 is the Yuan source point of kidneys and it activates the kidneys. CV-4 tonifies the kidneys Yang and Qi. BL-20 strengthens the spleen. BL-23 strengthens kidneys. CV-6 strengthens Qi. GV-3 and CV-8 ( do not needle ) activate kidneys Yang. Other points strengthen the lower burner and activate the kidneys. Medium level manipulation is used. Indirect moxibustion with salt is used on CV-8 and lower abdomen.

### <164> Frostbite

Frostbite is an emergency situation. Medical consultation is essential. The main treatment idea is to move blood to make the blood circulation on the local area. Bloodletting technique can activate the blood movement. Moxibustion can be applied to warm the local area and to increase the blood movement.

The main points : Ashi
The accompanying points :
For fingers : Ba xie ( Ex ), LI-4 ( He gu ), SI-6 ( Yang lao ), LI-10 ( Shou san li )
For toes : Ba feng ( Ex ), SP-6 ( San yin jiao ), ST-36 ( Zu san li ), GB-34 ( Yang ling quan )

The most injured area is the ashi point. The accompanying points are the Yang channel points that activate the movement of Qi and blood of the local area. Ba xie and Ba feng are the extra acupoints on the hands and feet that treat the frostbite of hands and feet. Ba xie is a group of points between the fingers. Ba feng is a group of points between the toes. SP-6 nourishes blood. Bloodletting technique is used on the local area and after that, moxibustion is used.

### <165> Gout

In TCM view, gout is damp heat on the local area. Medical consultation is essential. Damp heat is easily generated when the middle burner has problem and also through foods. The main treatment idea is to clear the heat, drain the dampness and regulate the Qi and blood of the local area.

The main points : ST-36 ( Zu san li ), SP-4 ( Gong sun ), SP-6 ( San yin jiao ), CV-4 ( Guan yuan ), GV-14 ( Da zhui ), LI-11 ( Qu chi ), SP-9 ( Yin ling quan )
The accompanying points : GB-34 ( Yang ling quan ), Ashi ( when there is not much pain ), LI-4 ( He gu ), GB-39 ( Xuan zhong ), Liv-3 ( Tai chong ), SP-10 ( Xue hai )

GV-14 clears the heat. CV-4 activates the lower burner to eliminate the dampness. ST-36 eliminates the dampness. GB-39 nourishes the bone marrow and kidneys to benefit the lower limbs where easily feels the pain. LI-4 and LI-11 clears the damp heat. GB-34 eliminates the dampness of the lower limbs. SP-6 eliminates the dampness. Liv-3 moves blood to relieve the pain and stagnation. Moxibustion is used. Strong manipulation is used on accompanying points.

### <166> Hemoptysis

Hemoptysis is an airway bleeding. There can be many kinds of causes and diseases. Medical consultation is essential. If those causes or original diseases are known, the treatment has be focused on those causes or diseases first. Here we focus on the how to diminish the bleeding from the airway. The main treatment idea is to clear the heat of the lung, regulate the Qi and blood of lung, eliminate the phlegm from the lung, move blood to stop the bleeding.

The main points : BL-17 ( Ge shu ), LI-11 ( Qu chi ), Lu-10 ( Yu ji ), Lu-5 ( Chi ze ), Lu-6 ( Kong zui ), ST-40 ( Feng long ), LI-2 ( Er jian )

The accompanying points : BL-12 ( Feng men ), ST-44 ( Nei ting ), BL-18 ( Gan shu ), BL-13 ( Fei shu ), CV-12 ( Zhong wan ), ST-36 ( Zu san li ), LI-16 ( Ju gu )

The special points of the lung channel are used. Lu-5 is the he sea point of lung. Lu-6 is the Xi-cleft point of the lung. Lu-10 clears the heat from the lung. LI-16 regulates the large intestine and lung. BL-12 eliminates the pathogenic wind from the lung. ST-40 transforms the phlegm from the lung. CV-12 benefits the lung. BL-17 and BL-18 move blood and preserve blood on liver to stop bleeding. BL-13 is the back shu point of lung. ST-36 regulates the movement of Qi and eliminates the dampness. Medium level manipulation is used. Treatment of the causing disease is necessary.

### <167> Hypertension – mild case

In TCM view, hypertension is related with heart, kidneys, liver and Qi. Medical consultation is essential. But not all hypertension shows the symptoms and that is why detail observation is needed to differentiate the patterns. There are many patterns and different cases in hypertension but in general, this prescription is used to calm the liver yang and to regulate the heart and kidneys and nourish the blood and yin. If any other syndromes or patterns are known, the treatment has to focus on those syndrome or patterns. If there is a disease that causes hypertension, it is necessary to treat that disease.

The main points : Liv-3 ( Tai chong ), GB-20 ( Feng chi ), LI-11 ( Qu chi ), Yin tang ( Ex ), GV-20 ( Bai hui ), ST-36 ( Zu san li ), GB-39 ( Xuan zhong ), An mian ( Ex )

The accompanying points : LI-4 ( He gu ), SP-6 ( San yin jiao ), CV-5 ( Shi men ), ST-9 ( Ren ying ), ST-40 ( Feng long ), PC-6 ( Nei guan ), K-3 ( Tai xi )

LI-11 is the He sea point of large intestine and it regulates the Qi of Yang ming and lowers the blood pressure. ST-36 regulates the movement of Qi. PC-6 is the luo connecting point of pericardium and it regulates the heart function. Yin tang is the extra acupoint that calms the mind and relieves the headache. GV-20 regulates the Qi and relieves the headache. GB-20 eliminates the wind and headache. GB-39 nourishes blood and Yin. ST-40 eliminates the phlegm and regulates the movement of Qi and blood. CV-5 strengthens the lower burner. An mian is the extra acupoint to treat the insomnia. ST-9 regulates the movement of Qi and blood and regulates the blood pressure. Strong manipulation is used. Moxibustion is used on ST-36 and GB-39

### <168> Hypertension – severe case

This is the severe case of hypertension and there is a danger of ACV or severe headache. Medical consultation is essential. It can be an emergency case too. The TCM treatment is to open the orifices, calm the wind and regulate the movement of Qi.

The main points : ST-36 ( Zu san li ), Liv-3 ( Tai chong ), GV-20 ( Bai hui ), LI-11 ( Qu chi ), Jing well points of hands and feet, GV-14 ( Da zhui ), GB-20 ( Feng chi ), ST-8 ( Tou wei ), Yin tang ( Ex ), Er jian ( Auricular acupuncture, top of the ear ) : bloodletting technique

The accompanying points : GB-7 ( Qu bin ), LI-4 ( He gu ), PC-6 ( Nei guan ), PC-5 ( Jian shi ), GB-21 ( Jian jing ), GB-39 ( Xuan zhong ), Ht-7 ( Shen men ), Liv-2 ( Xing jian ), Tai yang ( Ex ) : bloodletting technique, ST-40 ( Feng long ) : bloodletting technique

Jing well points of hands and feet unblock the connection between the Yin and Yang channels and can help prevent ACV ( but it is necessary to take the hypertension medication for emergency case ). ST-36 regulates the movement of Qi and blood. LI-11 lowers blood pressure. GV-14 clears the heat from the Yang channels. GV-20 opens orifices and relieves the headache and prevents ACV. Yin tang is the extra acupoint to eliminate the wind from head and calm the mind. GB-20 eliminates the wind from the head. GB-7 relieves the headache and eliminates the wind. PC-5 and PC-6 regulates the heart. GB-21 regulates the movement of Qi. Tai yang is the extra acupoint at the temporal region of the head. Bloodletting technique on Er jian, Tai yang or ST-40 regulates the movement of Qi and blood and eliminates the pathogen. GB-39 nourishes blood and yin to hold back the rising yang. Bloodletting technique is used on Jing well points. Strong manipulation is used. Moxibustions on ST-36, GB-39 and GV-20 are effective.

### <169> Hyperthyroidism

Hyperthyroidism is related with excess heat, rising liver yang. Medical consultation is essential. In TCM view eliminating the excess heat and liver yang is important.

The main points : Qi ying ( Ex ), LI-11 ( Qu chi ), Liv-2 ( Xing jian ), SP-6 ( San yin jiao ), Jia ji ( C3~C5 ), GB-20 ( Feng chi ), PC-5 ( Jian shi )

The accompanying points : PC-6 ( Nei guan ), SP-4 ( Gong sun ), GV-20 ( Bai hui ), LI-4 ( He gu )

For palpitations and insomnia : PC-7 ( Da ling ), Ht-7 ( Shen men ), An mian ( Ex )

For hot and red face : Tai yang ( Ex ) : bloodletting technique, Er jian ( Auricular acupuncture ) : bloodletting technique, Liv-2 ( Xing xian ), ST-44 ( Nei ting ), LI-4 ( He gu )

For protruded eyes : BL-2 ( Zan zhu ), Liv-3 ( Tai chong ), ST-2 ( Si bai )

For excessive sweat : Ht-6 ( Yin xi ), LI-4 ( He gu ), K-7 ( Fu liu )

PC-5 calms the fast heart rate. SP-6 nourishes Yin to hold back the rising Yang. Qi ying is the extra acupoint that treats the hyperthyroidism and the location is same with ST-10 ( Shui tu ). Jia ji ( C3~C5 ) are the extra acupoints that relieve the tension on the neck and regulate the Qi and blood. Other accompanying points and additional points can be added according to the situation and case patterns. Medium level manipulation is used.

### <170> Hypotension

Hypotension can be related with deficiency of Qi, emotional depression or fatigue etc. Medical consultation is essential. But not all hypotension shows the symptoms and that is why detail observation is needed to differentiate the patterns. Usual symptoms are dizziness or fatigue. The main TCM treatment idea is to strengthen the Qi and blood, activate the heart and kidneys.

The main points : GV-20 ( Bai hui ), GV-4 ( Guan yuan ), ST-9 ( Ren ying ), GV-25 ( Su liao ), GV-14 ( Da zhui ), K-7 ( Fu liu )

The accompanying points : GV-26 ( Shui gou ), Ht-7 ( Shen men ), SI-3 ( Hou xi ), PC-6 ( Nei guan ), Liv-3 ( Tai chong ), ST-36 ( Zu san li )

ST-9 regulates the blood pressure. PC-6 activates the heart function. GV-26 stimulates the heart to move more forcefully. Liv-3 activates the movement of heart. SI-3 strengthens kidneys and Qi. GV-25 stimulates the heart to move more forcefully. Ht-7 is the Yuan source point of heart and activates the heart. GV-14 regulates the all Yang channels. Soft manipulation is used.

### <171> Nocturnal sweating ( Night sweats )

Nocturnal sweating itself is not a disease but can be an indicator of underlying diseases. Medical consultation is essential. But not all nocturnal sweating means pathological. There can be many causes like menopause, anxiety, antidepression medications, low blood sugar, alcohol or drug etc. In TCM view, nocturnal sweating is a symptom of deficiency of Yin. The main treatment idea is to nourish the Yin and clear the heat from deficiency.

The main points : Ht-6 ( Yin xi ), BL-15 ( Xin shu ), K-7 ( Fu liu ), Lu-9 ( Tai yuan ), BL-13 ( Fei shu ), GV-12 ( Shen zhu ), CV-4 ( Guan yuan ), K-2 ( Ran gu )

The accompanying points : CV-6 ( Qi hai ), K-3 ( Tai xi ), BL-23 ( Shen shu ), GV-20 ( Bai hui ), ST-36 ( Zu san li ), BL-11 ( Da zhu ), Lu-5 ( Chi ze )

Ht-6 is the Xi cleft point of heart channel and it stops night sweating. BL-13 nourishes Yin of lung. GV-12 tonifies Yin with used together with other yin tonifying acupoints and strengthens the bone. BL-15 nourishes Yin of heart. BL-23 nourishes Yin of kidneys. BL-11 nourishes yin and strengthens bone. K-7 nourishes kidneys. The accompanying points can be added to increase the effects. The accompanying points are also nourishing the yin and strengthens the body. Soft manipulation is used. Moxibustion is used for chronic case.

### <172> Obesity

Obesity is a complicated case. Although it is not a disease, it causes many other serious problems like cirrhosis, heart attack, kidneys problem, hypertension, internal inflammation and even cancer. Medical consultation is essential. So treatment of obesity is very important to maintain the health and prevent the diseases. In TCM view, obesity has many different causes like deficiency of Qi, accumulation of phlegm and dampness, stomach heat, damp heat etc. It is difficult to show all prescriptions here. So the prescription shown here is through auricular acupuncture. Classical acupuncture prescription is complicated and it is better refer to a special reference book about treatment of obesity through classical acupuncture. Here we show you auricular acupuncture points. The main treatment idea is diminishing hunger and regulating hormones through auricular acupuncture acupoints.

Prescription 1 : rins, shen men, spleen, stomach, large intestine, mouth, thirst, endocrine, heart, abdomen

Prescription 2 : stomach, endocrine, large intestine, lower abdomen, esophagus, pancreas, mouth, hunger, abdomen, thirst

Prescription 3 : supra-renal, endocrine, subcortical, large intestine, uterus, mouth, ovaries, stomach, brain, testicle, hunger, thirst

### <173> Pancreatitis

Pancreatitis is an inflammation of pancreas. Medical consultation is essential. The main symptoms are abdominal pain, nausea, vomiting, fever or chills, rapid heartbeat and shortness of breath or jaundice. The main causes are alcohol or big gall stones. In TCM view, it is damp heat on the middle burner that causes the stagnation of Qi, pain and heat.

The main points : LI-11 ( Qu chi ), LI-2 ( Er jian ), BL-20 ( Pi shu ), Ashi on the back, BL-50 ( Wei cang ) on the left side, BL-22 ( San jiao shu ), SP-9 ( Yin ling quan ), SP-4 ( Gong sun )

The accompanying points : GV-12 ( Shen zhu ), SP-6 ( San yin jiao ), GV-14 ( Da zhui ), SP-2 ( Da du ), CV-12 ( Zhong wan ), ST-21 ( Liang men ) on left side, BL-17 ( Ge shu ), Cui shu ( Ex ), ST-36 ( Zu san li )

CV-12 eliminates the dampness and phlegm from the middle burner. ST-21 is the Xi-cleft point of stomach ( Yang ming channel ) to relieve the abdominal pain and heat. BL-20 eliminates the pathogen from pancreas. BL-22 regulates the triple burner. SP-4 is the luo connecting point of spleen channel to treat pancreas. The accompanying points are added to increase the effects of main points. Cui shu is the extra acupoints on the middle back, 1.5 cun lateral to the lower border of the spinous process of the eighth thoracic vertebra (T8). Cui shu is at the height of pancreas and it activates the function of pancreas. BL-17 moves blood and also activates the local area, pancreas. ST-36 eliminates the dampness. BL-50 is used for epigastric pain or abdominal distension. Needles are used for acute case and the moxibustion is used for chronic case.

### <174> Peritonitis

Peritonitis is an inflammation on the thin layer inside the abdomen. Medical consultation is essential. That is between the chest and the pelvis. The main causes are infection from bacteria or fungi. It can happen from cirrhosis or kidneys problems. The symptoms are belly pain or tenderness, fever, bloated abdomen, loss of appetite, vomiting or nausea, diarrhea, reduced quantity of urine, thirst, fatigue etc. The main treatment idea of acupuncture is to eliminate the pathogen, regulate the digestion, eliminate the dampness to diminish the inflammation.

The main points : BL-23 ( Shen shu ), BL-18 ( Gan shu ), SP-9 ( Yin ling quan ), CV-12 ( Zhong wan ), Liv-13 ( Zhang men ), CV-9 ( Shui fen ), BL-20 ( Pi shu ), ST-40 ( Feng long )
The accompanying points : LI-11 ( Qu chi ), ST-36 ( Zu san li ), CV-6 ( Qi hai ), ST-27 ( Da ju ), GB-34 ( Yang ling quan ), CV-3 ( Zhong ji ), GV-12 ( Shen zhu ), SP-6 ( San yin jjiao ), BL-25 ( Da chang shu )

BL-20 eliminates dampness and pathogen from spleen. BL-23 strengthens kidneys. BL-25 regulates the digestion system and removes the pathogen from abdomen. CV-12 eliminates the phlegm and regulates the digestion. CV-9 promotes urination and eliminates the dampness. CV-6 strengthens Qi. ST-27 relieves the abdominal pain. CV-3 promotes urination and relieves the pain. Liv-13 is used for all kinds of Zang organ problems. LI-11 clears the heat and inflammation. GB-34 eliminates dampness. GV-12 eliminates interior wind and strengthens the body. Medium level manipulation is used. Moxibustion can be used too.

### <175> Physical weakness

Physical weakness is deficiency of Qi and blood. Medical consultation is essential. The main treatment idea of TCM is to strengthens the Qi and blood. The main organs to treat is spleen and kidneys.

The main points : CV-6 ( Qi hai ) : moxibustion, GV-20 ( Bai hui ), GV-12 ( Shen zhu ), CV-4 ( Guan yuan ) : moxibustion, CV-5 ( Shi men ), ST-36 ( Zu san li ), K-7 ( Fu liu )

The accompanying points : BL-52 ( Zhi shi ), TB-2 ( Ye men ), CV-12 ( Zhong wan ), GV-4 ( Ming men ) : moxibustion, SI-3 ( Hou xi ), BL-23 ( Shen shu ) : moxibustion, BL-43 ( Gao huang ) : moxibustion

CV-4 strengthens Qi and blood, Yin and Yang. CV-5 and CV-6 strengthens Qi. ST-36 regulates spleen and stomach to increase the absorption of nutrition and generates Qi. GV-12 eliminates the internal wind and strengthens the body. GV-4 increases the kidneys Yang and warms the body. BL-23 strengthens kidneys. BL-52 nourishes kidneys essence. K-7 strengthens kidneys. CV-12 regulates the Qi on the middle burner to activate it. Moxibustion can be used. In case of children, moxibustion is not used on ST-36.

### <176> Pleurisy

This is an inflammation condition on pleura, the thin layers of tissue that separate lung from the chest wall. The patients experience chest pain when breathe, cough or sneeze, shortness of breath, cough or fever. Medical consultation is essential. The causes are viral infection, bacterial infection, fungal infection, lung cancer, pulmonary embolism, rib fracture, inherited diseases, medication, autoimmune disorder, tuberculosis etc. The main treatment idea is to clear the heat from the lung, eliminate the inflammation, phlegm and relieve the chest pain.

The main points : CV-12 ( Zhong wan ), Lu-10 ( Yu ji ), GV-12 ( Shen zhu ), BL-11 ( Da zhu ), Liv-14 ( Qi men ), SI-11 ( Tian zong ), Lu-7 ( Lie gue )

The accompanying points : LI-4 ( He gu ), LI-11 ( Qu chi ), SP-21 ( Da bao ), Ashi, PC-5 ( Xi men ), GB-36 ( Wai qiu ), GV-10 ( Ling tai ), ST-40 ( Feng long ), ST-36 ( Zu san li ), BL-17 ( Ge shu )

GV-12 clears the heat from the lung and relieves the cough. BL-11 relieves the cough. GV-10 relieves the cough. BL-17 removes stagnation of blood and SI-11 relieves the pain and calms the asthma. CV-12 eliminates the phlegm and regulates the movement of Qi on middle burner. Liv-14 removes Qi stagnation and liberates liver Qi. SP-21 relieves the chest pain. PC-5 is the Xi-cleft point of pericardium and relieves the chest pain. GB-36 is the Xi-cleft point and relieves the pain. Ashi point relieves the pain. Needles with strong manipulation are used for acute case. Moxibustion is used for chronic case.

<177> **Scrofula**

Scrofula is a serious condition that tuberculosis bacteria cause symptoms outside the lung including inflammation and irritated lymph nodes on the neck. Medical consultation is essential. The causes are tuberculosis bacteria. The main treatment idea in TCM is to eliminate the inflammation, clear the heat, nourish the lung, eliminate the phlegm, remove the Qi stagnation of liver and regulate the lung Qi.

The main points : SP-6 ( San yin jiao ), K-6 ( Zhao hai ), Lu-7 ( Lie que ), TB-10 ( Tian jing ), GV-14 ( Da zhui ), Zhou jian ( Ex ), Ashi, GB-21 ( Jian jiang ), Liv-3 ( Tai chong ), SP-10 ( Xue hai )

The accompanying points : GB-38 ( Yang fu ), ST-40 ( Feng long ), BL-23 ( Shen shu ), BL-13 ( Fei shu ), BL-43 ( Gao huang ), Liv-13 ( Zhang men ), GB-41 ( Zu lin qi ), TB-6 ( Zhi gou ), BL-17 ( Ge shu )

GV-14 clears the body heat. TB-10 is the special point for scrofula. Zhou jian is the extra acupoint located on the top of the ulnar olecranon when the elbow is flexed. Zhou jian is used for scrofula. Ashi point removes the mass. GB-21 regulates the movement of Qi. Liv-13 treats the Zang organs. To nourish lung and kidneys, BL-13, BL-23, K-6 and SP-6 are used. Liv-3, SP-10, BL-17 removes the stagnation of Qi and blood. ST-40 transforms the phlegm. GB and TB channels are used to treat the neck where those channels pass. Moxibustion is used on the local points or ashi.

### <178> Stomatitis

This is a condition of inflammation and redness on the oral mucosa. Medical consultation is essential. There are two kinds of stomatitis. One is herpes stomatitis ( cold sore ) and aphthous stomatitis ( canker sore ). The cause is infection. Because the oral mucosa is an expression of the situation of stomach, the treatment is focused on stomach and stomach channel. The main treatment idea is to eliminate the inflammation, regulate the stomach, clear the excess heat or heat from deficiency ( following the syndrome ), nourish the stomach and relieve the pain from the mouth.

The main points : LI-4 ( He gu ), ST-44 ( Nei ting ), ST-7 ( Xia guan ), SP-2 ( Da du ), CV-14 ( Ju que ), ST-36 ( Zu san li ), CV-12 ( Zhong wan ), BL-21 ( Wei shu )

The accompanying points : LI-10 ( Shou san li ), ST-34 ( Liang qiu ), LI-11 ( Qu chi ), K-7 ( Fu liu ), LI-2 ( Er jian ), LI-20 ( Ying xiang ), BL-23 ( Shen shu ), K-2 ( Ran gu )

ST-44 clears the heat on the stomach channel that passes the mouth and relieves pain. ST-34 is the Xi-cleft point of stomach channel and relieves the pain. ST-36 regulates the stomach and relieves the pain. Other points are used to treat and regulate the stomach. SP-2 is the Ying spring point to clears the heat from the spleen channel.

ST-4, LI-20, ST-5 and ST-7 are the local point to move Qi and blood of the local area and to relieve the pain. Strong manipulation is used.

### <179> Stupefaction (1) – blocking syndrome

This is the condition of being unable to think clearly because of being tired extremely, bored or from drug. Medical consultation is essential. The blocking syndrome is TCM name to describe the blocked situation when Qi and blood are blocked and does not flow well and the orifices are blocked and make the unclear consciousness. This is an excess syndrome ( pattern ). In TCM, the unclear consciousness is because of blocked orifices. The main treatment idea is to open the orifices and to awaken the consciousness and eliminate the stagnation.

The main points : PC-6 ( Nei guan ), LI-4 ( He gu ), GV-20 ( Bai hui ), Shi xuan ( Ex ), Liv-3 ( Tai chong ), GV26 ( Shui gou ), K-1 ( Yong quan )
The accompanying points : GV-14 ( Da zhui ), ST-40 ( Feng long ), GB-20 ( Feng chi ), Liv-2 ( Xing jian ), CV-12 ( Zhong wan )

GV-26 opens the orifices and awakens the consciousness. Shi xuan is the extra acupoint located at the ends of the each finger. Shi xuan opens orifices and used for the emergency cases. LI-4 and Liv-3 open the orifices and regulate the movement of Qi. GV-14 awakens the brain where the GV channel enters into. PC-6 opens the orifices. ST-40 transforms the phlegm that may block the orifices. K-1 is the emergency point to open the orifices and awaken the consciousness. Bloodletting technique is used on Shi xuan at first. Strong manipulation is used on other points.

### <180> Stupefaction (2) – collapsing syndrome

This is collapsing syndrome ( pattern ) of stupefaction and the cause is collapsing. Medical consultation is essential. Collapsing is TCM word that describes the situation when the patient loses the Qi, blood, Yin or Yang in a short time. For example, if the patient loses a lot of blood because of car accident, that is the collapse of blood. Collapse is a kind of deficiency but collapse is more severe than just deficiency. The main treatment idea is to tonify and warm the body.

The main points : CV-4 ( Guan yuan ), GV-25 ( Su liao ), Liv-3 ( Tai chong ), Lu-9 ( Tai yuan ), GV-20 ( Bai hui ), ST-36 ( Zu san li ), GV-4 ( Ming men )
The accompanying points : PC-8 ( Lao gong ), TB-2 ( Ye men ), K-7 ( Fu liu ), SI-3 ( Hou xi ), LI-4 ( He gu ), CV-6 ( Qi hai )

GV-20 tonifies the Qi and holds the Qi not to sink. CV-6 and CV-4 tonify the Qi, Yin and Yang. GV-25 awakens the consciousness. Lu-9 and K-7 tonify lung and kidneys. LI-4 and PC-8 help consciousness recovers. ST-36 tonifies Qi and regulates the movement of Qi. Mainly moxibustion is used. Needles with medium level manipulation are used on GV-25, Lu-9 and K-7.

### <181> Sunstroke, heliosis (1)

Sunstroke happens with excessive heat on body or exertional exercises. Medical consultation is essential. The patient's body temperature can increase more than 40.0 degree celsius. Sunstroke is an emergency case and life threatening. Usually the treatment is cooling the body. In acupuncture, the cooling methods and opening the orifices are used.

The main points : LI-4 ( He gu ), GV-26 ( Shui gou ), GV-14 ( Da zhui ), PC-6 ( Nei guan ), LI-11 ( Qu chi ), Liv-3 ( Tai chong )
The accompanying points : CV-12 ( Zhong wan ), GV-20 ( Bai hui ), SP-4 ( Gong sun ), ST-36 ( Zu san li ), ST-43 ( Xian gu )

GV-14, LI-11 and LI-4 cool the body heat. ST-43 regulates the stomach and calms the nausea. Liv-3 activates the heart beats to recuperate. ST-36 tonifies Qi. PC-6 opens orifices and maintains the heart function and relieves the nausea or vomit. CV-12 eliminates the phlegm and regulates the middle burner to treat the nausea and vomit. SP-4 nourishes Yin and blood and regulates the spleen and stomach. Strong manipulation is used.

### <182> Sunstroke, heliosis (2)

Sunstroke happens with excessive heat on body or exertional exercises. Medical consultation is essential. The patient's body temperature can increase more than 40.0 degree celsius. Sunstroke is an emergency case and life threatening. Usually the treatment is cooling the body. In acupuncture, the cooling methods and opening the orifices are used.

The main points : K-7 ( Fu liu ), K-1 ( Yong quan ), Shi xuan ( Ex ) or Jing well points of hands, GV-26 ( Shui gou ), PC-3 ( Qu ze ), Jin jin ( Ex ), Yu ye ( Ex )

The accompanying points : BL-57 ( Cheng shan ), ST-36 ( Zu san li ), BL-40 ( Wei zhong ), GV-20 ( Bai hui ), PC-8 ( Lao gong ), SP-6 ( San yin jiao )

GV-26 awakens the consciousness. Shi xuan is the extra acupoint located at the ends of the each finger. Shi xuan is an emergency acupoint to open the orifices. Jing well points of hands have the same meaning with Shi xuan. PC-3 helps recuperate the heart beat and lung functions. BL-40 clears the blood heat. GV-20 tonifies Qi and holds Qi not to sink. PC-8 opens the orifices. K-1 is the emergency acupoint to awaken the consciousness. BL-57 relieves the body spasm. Jin jin and Yu ye are the extra acupoints located under the tongue. Jin jin and Yu ye clears the body heat rapidly and increase the body fluids. Bloodletting technique is used on Shi xuan, PC-3 and BL-40. Strong manipulations are used on other points.

### <183> Syncope, faint

Syncope is fainting or passing out. Medical consultation is essential. The main causes are usually sudden lack of blood flow into brain. The main treatment idea of acupuncture is regulating the heart and kidneys, tonifying Qi and blood and opening the orifices to awaken the consciousness.

The main points : K-1 ( Yong quan ), PC-9 ( Zhong chong ), ST-36 ( Zu san li ), GV-26 ( Shui gou ), GV-20 ( Bai hui ), Ht-9 ( Shao chong )

The accompanying points : SI-3 ( Hou xi ) to PC-8 ( Lao gong ), ST-36 ( Zu san li ), PC-6 ( Nei guan ), Lu-11 ( Shao shang )

GV-26 opens the orifices to awaken the consciousness. PC-9 activates the heart functions and also opens the orifices. Ht-9 activates the heart beats. ST-36 tonifies and regulates the Qi and blood. Lu-11 is the Jing well point of lung channel and used for emergency case. LI-4 opens the orifices and regulates the Qi. SI-3 activates kidneys. PC-8 activates heart beats. K-1 is used for emergency cases and awakens the consciousness. First, needle GV-26 with strong manipulation. Bloodletting technique is used on PC-9 and Ht-9.

### <184> Total exhaustion (1)

Total exhaustion can be an emergency case. Medical consultation is essential. Proper absorption of nutrients, ions and liquid is necessary. In Acupuncture, the main treatment idea is tonifying Qi and blood, opening orifices to make clear consciousness.

The main points : PC-6 ( Nei guan ), CV-4 ( Guan yuan ) : moxibustion, GV-25 ( Su liao ), GV-20 ( Bai hui ) : moxibustion

The accompanying points : GV-26 ( Shui gou ), PC-9 ( Zhong chong ), K-1 ( Yong quan ), ST-36 ( Zu san li ), CV-12 ( Zhong wan ) : moxibustion

GV-25 awakens the consciousness and makes Qi ascend. PC-6 opens orifices. GV-26 opens orifices and makes Qi ascend. PC-9 opens orifices and activates the heart beats. K-1 is an emergency acupoint to awaken the brain and tonify kidneys Qi. ST-36 tonifies Qi and regulates the Qi movement. Soft manipulation is used.

### <185> Total exhaustion (2)

Total exhaustion can be an emergency case. Medical consultation is essential. Proper absorption of nutrients, ions and liquid is necessary. In Acupuncture, the main treatment idea is tonifying Qi and blood, opening orifices to make clear consciousness.

The main points : GV-26 ( Shui gou ), CV-8 ( Shen que ) : moxibustion, CV-4 ( Guan yuan ) : moxibustion, GV-20 ( Bai hui ) : moxibustion

The accompanying points : K-1 ( Yong quan ), CV-6 ( Qi hai ) : moxibustion, ST-36 ( Zu san li ) : moxibustion, GV-4 ( Ming men ) : moxibustion

GV-20 tonifies Qi and holds Qi not to sink. CV-8 ( moxibustion ) tonifies Yang of kidneys and warms the body. CV-6 and CV-4 tonifies Qi and blood. ST-36 tonifies Qi and GV-4 warms the body and activates the kidneys Yang. Moxibustion is used. Indirect moxibustion is used on CV-8.

### <186> Tympanites

This is the accumulation of gas in the gastrointestinal tract. Medical consultation is essential. The patients experience bloating, distention and discomfort. There can be many different causes but in acupuncture the main treatment idea is regulating the gastrointestinal tract to eliminate the gas and make the digestive system function normally.

The main points : Liv-3 ( Tai chong ), LI-10 ( Shou san li ), CV-4 ( Guan yuan ), Liv-13 ( Zhang men ), SP-6 ( San yin jiao ), ST-37 ( Shang ju xu ), CV-6 ( Qi hai ), SP-14 ( Fu jie ), ST-36 ( Zu san li )

The accompanying points : BL-22 ( San jiao shu ), ST-40 ( Feng long ), CV-9 ( Shui fen ), K-9 ( Zhu bin ), ST-25 ( Tian shu ), K-14 ( Si man )

In case of neural ( mental ) cause : GV-20 ( Bai hui ), Ht-7 ( Shen men ), PC-6 ( Nei guan )

Mainly the acupoints on the stomach and large intestine channels are used. SP-6 eliminates the dampness and activates the spleen. LI-10 strengthens spleen and stomach and also eliminates the dampness. ST-36 activates stomach and regulates the Qi not to accumulate the gas on the gastrointestinal tract. K-9, SP-14, CV-6 and K-14 are the local acupoints to regulate and move the Qi on the local area. The accompanying points are the local points around the abdomen and the points that activate the Qi and movement of heart. Medium level manipulation is used.

### <187> Vertigo

In TCM view, vertigo is a kind of wind generated from the deficiency or also from excess syndrome. Medical consultation is essential. And also phlegm on the middle burner can block the movement of Qi from spleen to brain and makes vertigo. When liver yang rises and generates the wind, the patient will experience vertigo. The main treatment idea is to calm the wind, nourish the yin or blood to hold the wind back and to transform the phlegm from the middle burner.

The main points : GB-20 ( Feng chi ), CV-4 ( Guan yuan ), LI-4 ( He gu ), GV-20 ( Bai hui ), PC-6 ( Nei guan ), SP-6 ( San yin jiao ), ST-40 ( Feng long )

The accompanying points : GV-18 ( Qiang jian ), CV-12 ( Zhong wan ), GB-8 ( Shuai gu ), ST-36 ( Zu san li ), TB-17 ( Yi feng ), SI-19 ( Ting gong ), Liv-3 ( Tai chong ), Yin tang ( Ex )

GB-20 calms the wind. GV-20 holds the Qi in the head and treats vertigo. Yin tang is the extra acupoint to calm the mind and treats vertigo. LI-4 and Liv-3 regulate the movement of Qi. ST-36 makes the Qi descend to diminish the wind. ST-36 has the function of strengthening the Qi but in case of vertigo because of deficiency of blood in brain, it is better use other points to strengthen the Qi rather than ST-36. It is because ST-36 activates the movement of blood in digestive tract and make the blood flow more in the digestive tract and the brain possibly be in lack of blood and it will delay the time to be recover from the vertigo. In ancient classic of acupuncture, ST-36 is sometimes used for blood deficiency but that is not the case of blood deficiency in brain and we can consider the function of ST-36. GV-18 eliminates the wind in the head and treats vertigo. ST-40 regulates the movement of Qi and eliminates the phlegm. SP-6 nourishes Yin. GB-8 eliminates the wind from the head. TB-17 eliminates the wind. SI-19 treats the ear to have clear balance perception. Medium level manipulation is used.

### <188> Vomiting blood, hematemesis

Vomiting blood is not a good sign. Medical consultation is essential. The patient has to go to the hospital and do the medical exam because there can be serious illness as a cause. In this treatment scheme, the treatment is focused on stopping the bleeding. The main treatment idea is cooling the blood, warm the abdomen.

The main points : BL-17 ( Ge shu ), PC-6 ( Nei guan ), SP-10 ( Xue hai ), BL-23 ( Shen shu ), GV-4 ( Ming men ), K-7 ( Fu liu ), Ht-6 ( Yin xi ), SP-6 ( San yin jiao )

The accompanying points : GB-34 ( Yang ling quan ), LI-11 ( Qu chi ), Liv-2 ( Xing jian ), Ht-8 ( Shao fu ), Lu-5 ( Chi ze ), K-10 ( Yin gu ), TB-8 ( San yang luo )

K-10 and K-7 is to strengthen Yang of the kidneys to warm the stomach. Lu-5 and PC-6 regulates the movement of blood. GV-4 warms the stomach. BL-23 tonifies the kidneys. Ht-6 regulates heart to control the movement of blood. TB-8 regulates the passage of Qi and blood. Liv-2 and Ht-8 are Ying spring points to cool the heat in the liver and the heart. GB-34 eliminates the dampness and stagnation of Qi in Shao yang. Treatment of the causing disease is necessary. Medium level manipulation is used.

# | 18 |

# Liver and gall bladder

**<189> Cholecystitis, inflammation of gall bladder**

The main treatment idea is eliminating the heat pathogen in the shao yang channel. Medical consultation is essential.

The main points : GB-24 ( Ri yue ), GB-43 ( Xia xi ), GB-34 ( Yang ling quan ), Liv-14 ( Qi men ) on the right side, BL-19 ( Dan shu ), GB-40 ( Qiu xu ), ST-21 ( Liang men ) on the right side, BL-18 ( Gan shu ) on the right side, CV-12 ( Zhong wan ), Liv-2 ( Xing jian ), Dan nang xue ( Ex )

The accompanying points : GV-12 ( Shen zhu ), Liv-3 ( Tai chong ), LI-11 ( Qu chi ), Lu-6 ( Kong zui ), CV-14 ( Ju que ), SI-11 ( Tian zong ) on the right side, LI-4 ( He gu ), ST-40 ( Feng long ), BL-48 ( Yang gang ), GB-36 ( Wai qiu )

Dan nang xue is the extra acupoint for gall bladder problems. It clears the heat and drains damp. The location of Dan nang xue is a tender spot 1 ~ 2 cun below GB-34. GB-34 is the lower hui meeting point of GB channel and clears the heat of Shao yang. GB-36 clears the heat of Shao yang. GB-24 is the front mu point of gall bladder to eliminate the heat from gall bladder. BL-19 is the back shu point of gall bladder. BL-48 eliminates the heat from gall bladder. SI-11 is the local point. CV-12 regulates the Qi and eliminates the dampness.

CV-14 is the local point. Liv-14 is the local point to eliminate the stagnation of liver Qi. ST-21 is the Xi-cleft point and eliminates the pain. BL-18 eliminates the stagnation and pain on the gall bladder and liver. GV-12 nourishes body and Lu-6 is the Xi-cleft point of lung and treats fever. Reducing manipulation is used mainly on the main points. The accompanying points are used selectively.

### <190> Cholelithiasis, gall stone

Gall stones are easily formed with greasy foods or meat products. There are genetic causes too. Medical consultation is essential. In TCM view, gall stones are a kind of damp heat. The main treatment idea is to eliminate the damp heat from the gall bladder. Many other organs are related with this problem.

The main points : Dan nang xue ( Ex ), GB-43 ( Xia xi ), BL-18 ( Gan shu ), GB-24 ( Ri yue ) on the right side, Liv-3 ( Tai chong ), GB-36 ( Wai qiu ), BL-19 ( Dan shu ), ST-21 ( Liang men ), GB-40 ( Qiu xu ), Liv-14 ( Qi men ) on the right side, GB-34 ( Yang ling quan )

The accompanying points : Liv-2 ( Xing jian ), CV-12 ( Zhong wan ), SP-16 ( Fu ai ), Lu-6 ( Kong zui ), LI-4 ( He gu ), BL-50 ( Wei cang ), PC-4 ( Xi men ), SI-11 ( Tian zong ) on the right side

Liver has to be treated together because liver generates the bile that is preserved in gall bladder and also in TCM view, liver is the internal partner of gall bladder. Dan nang xue is the extra acupoint for gall bladder problems. It clears the heat and drains damp. The location of Dan nang xue is a tender spot 1 ~ 2 cun below GB-34. Liv-14 is the front mu point of liver. GB-24 is the front mu point of gall bladder. ST-21, CV-12 and SP-16 relieve the pain on the middle burner. GB-36 eliminates the damp heat from gall bladder channel. GB-40 is the Yuan source point of gall bladder and it eliminates the damp heat from the gall bladder. BL-19 is the back shu point of gall bladder. BL-18 is the back shu point of liver. BL-50 relieves the pain in the epigastric region. GB-34 eliminates the damp heat. PC-4 eliminates the chest pain. SI-11 eliminates the local pain. Lu-6 is the Xi-cleft point of lung and it reduces the chest pain. This prescription is for the outbreak of acute pain for gall stone. If the pain is severe, it is necessary to do surgery. Strong manipulation is used. The accompanying points can be used selectively.

### <191> Cirrhosis

Cirrhosis is life threatening if the process is advanced. There are alcoholic cirrhosis and non-alcoholic cirrhosis. Medical consultation is essential. Proper diet and exercise are necessary. The main treatment idea is to eliminate the dampness, regulate the liver and activate the digestion and metabolism. The treatment has to be done on liver, gall bladder and spleen and stomach because the dampness is generated from middle burner.

The main points : CV-12 ( Zhong wan ), ST-36 ( Zu san li ), Liv-14 ( Qi men ), BL-18 ( Gan shu ), Liv-3 ( Tai chong ), Ashi points, SP-10 ( Xue hai ), GB-34 ( Yang ling quan ), SI-11 ( Tian zong ), ST-40 ( Feng long ) : bloodletting technique

The accompanying points : SP-6 ( San yin jiao ), SP-9 ( Yin ling quan ), Liv-2 ( Xing jian ), GV-12 ( Shen zhu ), BL-19 ( Dan shu ), GV-9 ( Zhi yang ), Liv-8 ( Qu quan ), CV-9 ( Shui fen )

Liv-14 is the front mu point of liver and BL-18 is the back shu point of liver. Those points eliminate the dampness from the liver and gall bladder and regulate them. CV-12 activates spleen and stomach to eliminate the dampness and phlegm. Liv-3 is the Yuan source point of liver. GV-12 strengthens the body and eliminates the heat. BL-19 is the back shu point of gall bladder. SI-11 regulates the local area and relieves the pain. GB-34 and SP-6 eliminate the dampness. GV-9 eliminates the damp from the liver and gall bladder. The moxibustion is used. 5-7 times for one session. This treatment can be used for the initial and middle stage of cirrhosis. Medication and moxibustion must be used together. If the patient has ascites, this treatment does not work well.

### <192> Hepatitis

There are different types of hepatitis depending on the types of infections. Medical consultation is essential. In TCM view, the treatment is to eliminate the damp heat, heat or cold damp and regulate the liver, gall bladder and spleen. The main pathogen is damp.

The main points : PC-6 ( Nei guan ), SP-10 ( Xue hai ), GB-34 ( Yang ling quan ), Jing well points of hands, GV-28 ( Yin jiao ), LI-11 ( Qu chi ), BL-18 ( Gan shu ), ST-36 ( Zu san li ), BL-20 ( Pi shu ), TB-6 ( Zhi gou )

The accompanying points : Liv-4 ( Zhong feng ), LI-4 ( He gu ), GV-9 ( Zhi yang ), Liv-3 ( Tai chong ), SP-9 ( Yin ling quan ), BL-19 ( Dan shu )

The Jing well points of hands are used to open the orifices and to eliminate the heat pathogen. GV-28 is the special point for clearing the heat of hepatitis. GV-9 eliminates the damp heat. BL-18 is the back shu point of liver. BL-20 is the back shu point of spleen. GB-34 eliminates the damp heat. ST-36 eliminates damp. BL-19 is the back shu point of gall bladder. TB-6 opens the TB channel to eliminate the damp. PC-6 regulates the liver, Qi and also regulates the middle burner to eliminate the damp. Liv-4 and Liv-3 eliminate the damp from the liver. Bleeding method is used on Jing well points and GV28 ( Yin jiao ). Strong manipulation is used to eliminate the pathogen ( this way is for acute and excess syndrome )

### <193> Jaundice

Usually there are three kinds of Jaundice in TCM like damp heat type, cold damp type, and deficiency type. Medical consultation is essential. Depending on the syndrome and patterns you can modify the prescription. The main idea of treatment is to eliminate the damp and regulate the liver, gall bladder and spleen. If the syndrome is cold, you can add the warming method. If the syndrome is heat, you can add the clearing method. If it is deficiency, you can add tonifying method.

The main points : LI-11 ( Qu chi ), GB-34 ( Yang ling quan ), BL-19 ( Dan shu ), Liv-3 ( Tai chong ), BL-17 ( Ge shu ), BL-20 ( Pi shu ), GV-9 ( Zhi yang ), CV-12 ( Zhong wan ), SP-6 ( San yin jiao ), Liv-14 ( Qi men )

The accompanying points : Dan nang xue ( Ex ), Jing well points of the hands, GB-20 ( Feng chi ), ST-21 ( Liang men ), Liv-14 ( Zhang men ), GV-12 ( Shen zhu ), Liv-8 ( Qu quan ), BL-18 ( Gan shu ), ST-36 ( Zu san li )

GV-9 clears the body heat. BL-17 is the hui meeting point of blood and detoxifies the blood, eliminates the blood heat and stagnation. Dan nang xue is the extra acupoint for gall bladder problems. It clears the heat and drains damp. The location of Dan nang xue is a tender spot 1 ~ 2 cun below GB-34. BL-19 is the back shu point of gall bladder to eliminate the damp. BL-20 eliminates the damp. Liv-8, Liv-3 and SP-6 eliminate the damp from the liver and spleen. ST-21 relieves the pain and eliminates the damp from the middle burner. Liv-14 is the front mu point of liver and eliminates the damp from liver. Bleeding on the Jing well points can clear the heat. Liv-14 is the hui meeting point of Zang organ and treats the liver and spleen. The bleeding method is used on the Jing well points. The strong manipulation is used for other points to eliminate the pathogens ( this prescription is for excess syndrome ).

# | 19 |

# Men's health

<194> **Benign prostatic hyperplasia**

With aging process, prostatic hyperplasia is very common. Mental consultation is essential. In TCM view, the liver channel passes the sexual organ and the treatment is focused on regulating liver channel and eliminating the damp. The acupoints that moves Qi of liver channel are commonly used. Also activating urination method is used to relieve the urination difficulty.

The main points : K-11 ( Heng gu ), ST-9 ( Shui fen ), BL-32 ( Zhong liao ), BL-32 ( Ci liao ), CV-3 ( Zhong ji ), BL-18 ( Gan shu ), K-10 ( Yin gu ), SP-9 ( Yin ling quan ), SP-6 ( San yin jiao ), CV-2 ( Qu gu ), Liv-5 ( Li gou ), Long men ( Ex )

The accompanying points : Liv-8 ( Qu quan ), K-7 ( Fu liu ), BL-23 ( Shen shu ), GV-4 ( Ming men ), ST-30 ( Qi chong ), Lu-7 ( Lie que ), SP-8 ( Di ji ), BL-39 ( Wei yang ), SP-15 ( Da heng ), SP-10 ( Xue hai ), Liv-3 ( Tai chong )

CV-3 and CV-2 is the special point to activate the urination and also to relieve the pain. They have a very good effect on prostate and are the main points for prostate problem. K-11 regulates the local area of prostate. BL-18 is the back shu point of liver. BL-23 is the back shu point of kidneys to facilitate the urination. Liv-5 is the luo connecting point of liver channel and it regulates the urine flows. BL-32 is on the sacral region and regulates the local region of prostate. K-10 regulates the local area of prostate. Liv-8 eliminates the damp from the liver channel and prostate. SP-6 eliminates the damp. BL-39 activates the urination and eliminates the damp. The accompanying points are regulating the local area of prostate and increase the kidneys Yang to activate the urination. Long men is the extra acupoint located at the lower edge of the pubic bone on the conception vessel (Ren mai). Long men has a very good effect on difficulty in urination. Medium level manipulation is used. The points are used selectively. The moxibustion and needles can be used together. Long term treatment is necessary.

### <195> Erectile dysfunction (1)

Erectile dysfunction has complex and various causes like emotional problem, smoking, alcohol, fatigue, mental stress or depression, blood circulation problem etc. Medical consultation is essential. But in TCM view, the organs related are liver, kidneys and Qi or Yang. The prescription introduced here is only for the symptom itself and if any causes are known, the treatment of those causes has to be added. The main treatment idea of this prescription is to increase the Yang of kidneys that is the most common treatment.

The main points : ST-36 ( Zu san li ), SP-8 ( Di ji ), SP-4 ( Gong sun ), GV-4 ( Ming men ), CV-4 ( Guan yuan ), TB-2 ( Ye men ), SP-6 ( San yin jiao ), BL-32 ( Ci liao ), BL-23 ( Shen shu ), CV-2 ( Qu gu )
The accompanying points : CV-6 ( Qi hai ), Liv-3 ( Tai chong ), SI-3 ( Hou xi ), K-6 ( Zhao hai ), ST-29 ( Gui lai ), K-2 ( Ran gu )
In case of mental stress : add GV-20 ( Bai hui ), PC-6 ( Nei guan )

BL-32 activates the kidneys Yang, Qi and blood circulation on the pelvis. GV-4 increases the Kidneys Yang. ST-36 strengthens the Qi. CV-4 nourishes kidneys and lower burner. BL-23 strengthens the kidneys. SP-6 nourishes the blood and eliminates the dampness. The accompanying points are the local points to increase the Qi or nourish the kidneys and liver. Medium level manipulation is used. The points are used selectively. Once a day or once for two days treatment. In chronic case, the moxibustion is used 5-7 times for a session.

### <196> Erectile dysfunction (2)

Erectile dysfunction has complex and various causes like emotional problem, smoking, alcohol, fatigue, mental stress or depression, blood circulation problem etc. Medical consultation is essential. But in TCM view, the organs related are liver, kidneys and Qi or Yang. The prescription introduced here is only for the symptom itself and if any causes are known, the treatment of those causes has to be added. The main treatment idea of this prescription is to increase the Yang of kidneys that is the most common treatment.

The main points : Long men ( Ex ), SP-6 ( San yin jiao ), CV-6 ( Qi hai ), CV-2 ( Qu gu ), Liv-5 ( Li gou ), Ht-7 ( Shen men )

The accompanying points : BL-23 ( Shen shu ), CV-3 ( Zhong ji ), GV-4 ( Ming men ), CV-4 ( Guan yuan ), BL-52 ( Zhi shi ), SP-8 ( Di ji )

You can refer to the erectile dysfunction (1) for the point explanations. Some different points are used in this second prescription. Long men is the extra acupoint located at the lower edge of the pubic bone on the conception vessel (Ren mai). Liv-5 is the luo connecting point of liver channel and this point has a good effect on urinary problems or sexual problems. In this second prescription, treatment of heart is added like Ht-7 that calms the mind. If the cause of erectile dysfunction is emotional or related with mental stress, Ht-7 can be added. The soft manipulation is used. The moxibustion is used for the chronic cases.

### <197> Male infertility

Male infertility is mainly related with the low activity and numbers of sperms. Medical consultation is essential. This prescription will help increase the sperm activity and its numbers. In TCM view, low sperm activity is deficiency of kidneys, liver and Qi. So the main treatment idea is to tonify kidneys, liver and Qi.

The main points : ST-27 ( Da ju ), K-7 ( Fu liu ), BL-53 ( Bao huang ), ST-36 ( Zu san li ), BL-23 ( Shen shu ), CV-4 ( Guan yuan ) : good to use moxibustion, CV-12 ( Zhong wan ), GV-4 ( Ming men ), SP-6 ( San yin jiao )

The accompanying points : ST-28 ( Shui dao ), BL-31 ( Shang liao ), BL-27 ( Xiao chang shu ), Liv-5 ( Li gou ), Zi gong ( Ex, Note : Male also has Zi gong point ), ST-29 ( Gui lai ), LI-4 ( He gu ), Liv-3 ( Tai chong ), K-3 ( Tai xi )

In case of mental stress : add GV-20 ( Bai hui ), Liv-2 ( Xing jian ), Ht-7 ( Shen men )

The main points are tonifying the kidneys, Qi and nourishing the body. The accompanying points are nourishing liver and blood. Zi gong is the extra acupoint. Zi gong is not just on the female body but also is on the male body too. The location is 3 cun lateral to CV-3 ( Zhong ji ). The function of Zi gong is increasing the sexual power for man and woman. The moxibustion is more effective than needles. Moxibustion is used 5-7 times for a session. The points are used selectively. The treatment can be done once for 3 days. Long term treatment is necessary.

### <198> Nocturnal emission

Nocturnal emission is a symptom of losing sperms during night time. Medical consultation is essential. Nocturnal emission is a serious problem from men. If it becomes chronic, the men can become seriously exhausted and the fatigue will continue. It makes the body more and more deficient and the treatment becomes more difficult. Nocturnal emission has to be treated early. In TCM view, nocturnal emission is deficiency of kidneys, liver and Qi or damp heat and emotional issue. The main treatment idea here is to tonify the body.

The main points : GV-20 ( Bai hui ), CV-3 ( Zhong ji ), K-6 ( Zhao hai ), CV-4 ( Guan yuan ) : good to use moxibustion, SP-6 ( San yin jiao ), BL-23 ( Shen shu ), BL-15 ( Xin shu ), SP-8 ( Di ji )

The accompanying points : Liv-2 ( Xing jian ), ST-36 ( Zu san li ), GV-4 ( Ming men ) : good to use moxibustion, PC-5 ( Jian shi ), K-2 ( Ran gu ), Liv-8 ( Qu quan )

In case of mental stress and fear : add PC-6 ( Nei guan ) or TCM herbal medicine

The main points are to tonify kidneys Yang and liver. PC-5 and BL-15 calm the mind. K-2 eliminates the heat from the lower burner. BL-23 nourishes the kidneys. The medium level manipulation is used. The treatment is applied once for 2 days. The moxibustion is used for the chronic cases.

### <199> Orchitis

Orchitis is an inflammation of testicle. Bacterial or viral infections are the main causes or some causes are unknown. Medical consultation is essential. Usually sexual activity can transmit this infection. In TCM view damp heat on the liver channel is the main syndrome ( pattern ) and if the case becomes chronic, the syndrome changes into deficiency. The main treatment idea of this prescription is to clear the damp heat on the liver channel.

The main points : SP-1 ( Yin bai ), SP-9 ( Yin ling quan ), Liv-1 ( Da dun ), CV-3 ( Zhong ji ), Liv-5 ( Li gou ), ST-30 ( Qi chong ), Liv-3 ( Tai chong )

The accompanying points : ST-36 ( Zu san li ), Liv-2 ( Xing jian ), ST-29 ( Gui lai ), CV-4 ( Guan yuan ), BL-23 ( Shen shu ), Du yin ( Ex ), SP-6 ( San yin jiao )

The bleeding method can be used for Liv-1 and SP-1 to clear the heat from the liver channel and lower burner. SP-9, CV-3, ST-29 and SP-6 eliminate the dampness from the lower burner. Du yin is the extra acupoint to move blood and stop pain. The location is on plantar side of second toe, on the center of the distal interphalangeal skin crease. Other accompanying points are eliminating the pathogens from the lower burner and especially from the liver channel. The strong manipulation is used. The points are used selectively.

### <200> Premature ejaculation

The main causes of premature ejaculation are deficiency of kidneys, spleen Qi, liver qi stagnation, damp heat etc. Medical consultation is essential. The main treatment idea in this prescription is nourishing the liver and kidneys.

The main points : Liv-2 ( Xing jian ), CV-2 ( Qu gu ), CV-3 ( Zhong ji ), CV-4 ( Guan yuan ), SP-6 ( San yin jiao ), BL-32 ( Ci liao ), K-2 ( Ran gu )
The accompanying points : K-3 ( Tai xi ), ST-29 ( Gui lai ), ST-36 ( Zu san li ), Liv-3 ( Tai chong ), CV-6 ( Qi hai ), ST-30 ( Qi chong ), SP-9 ( Yin ling quan )
In case of mental stress : GV-20 ( Bai hui ), PC-6 ( Nei guan ), Ht-7 ( Shen men )

The main and accompanying points are for nourishing kidneys and liver, regulating the Qi and eliminating the damp heat from the lower burner. The medium level manipulation is used. Moxibustion is used on CV-3. Treatment can be done once for 2 days

### <201> Prostatitis

Prostatitis is an inflammation of prostate. The bacterial infection is the main causes but not always. Some causes are unknown. Medical consultation is essential. In TCM view, the damp heat is the cause for the acute cases and deficiency patterns are for the chronic cases. The main treatment idea of this prescription is to eliminate the damp heat from the lower burner and liver channel.

The main points : Liv-5 ( Li gou ), CV-2 ( Qu gu ), CV-4 ( Guan yuan ), BL-23 ( Shen shu ), Long men ( Ex ), SP-6 ( San yin jiao ), CV-3 ( Zhong ji ), Liv-3 ( Tai chong ), BL-28 ( Pang guan shu )

The accompanying points : ST-28 ( Shui dao ), GV-20 ( Bai hui ), LI-11 ( Qu chi ), SP-9 ( Yin ling quan ), Liv-8 ( Qu quan ), ST-29 ( Gui lai ), Liv-2 ( Xing jian )

The points are to eliminate the damp heat from the lower burner and liver channel. To eliminate the dampness from the lower burner, it is good to promote urination. Long men is the extra acupoint to promote the urination and to eliminate the dampness from the lower burner. The location of Long men is at the lower border of the pubic bone on the conception vessel ( Ren mai ). The medium or strong level manipulation is used everyday or once for 2 days.

### <202> Sexual insensitivity, frigidity

Sexual insensitivity is a complex symptom because there can be various causes. Qi deficiency or stagnation, damp heat, damp coldness or mental stress can be the main causes. Medical consultation is essential. The main treatment idea in this prescription is to regulate the liver channel to eliminate the pathogens and increase the Qi and kidneys to have more sexual sensitivity.

The main points : ST-36 ( Zu san li ), Long men ( Ex ), BL-17 ( Ge shu ), GV-20 ( Bai hui ), Liv-8 ( Qu quan ), Liv-1 ( Da dun ), CV-3 ( Zhong ji )

The accompanying points : K-12 ( Da he ), BL-32 ( Ci liao ), BL-23 ( Shen shu ), GV-12 ( Shen zhu ), BL-27 ( Xiao chang shu ), Ht-8 ( Shao fu ) : tonify in case of cold syndrome

In case of mental stress : PC-6 ( Nei guan ), Ht-7 ( Shen men ), Si shen cong ( Ex )

Liv-1 eliminates the pathogens from the liver channel. Liv-8 eliminates the dampness from the liver channel and also nourishes the liver. Long men is the extra acupoint and the location is on the lower border of the pubic bone on the conception vessel ( Ren mai ). It eliminates the dampness and promotes the urination. BL-27 and BL-23 eliminates the pathogens from the pelvis and also tonify the kidneys Yang to increase the sexual insensitivity. GV-20 increases the Qi and also relieves the mental stress. GV-12 nourishes the body. BL-17 increases the blood circulation. Medium level manipulation is used.

# | 20 |

# Nerve problems

### <203> Facial nerve paralysis

The main origin of this symptom is the damaged 7th cranial nerve ( facial nerve ). Medical consultation is essential. The main causes can be infection, trauma or stroke. In TCM, the main treatment idea is to eliminate the wind from the head and face, regulate the local area and activate the blood circulation.

The main points : ST-4 ( Di cang ), LI-11 ( Qu chi ), GB-20 ( Feng chi ), ST-36 ( Zu san li ), LI-4 ( He gu ), ST-37 ( Shang ju xu ), ST-6 ( Jia che ), TB17 ( Yi feng ), ST-2 ( Si bai ), GB-14 ( Yang bai ), Qian zheng ( Ex )

The accompanying points : Tai yang ( Ex ), Liv-3 ( Tai chong ) ST-44 ( Nei ting ), Jia cheng jiang ( Ex ), ST-7 ( Xia guan ), GV-26 ( Shui gou ), GB-31 ( Feng shi )

GB-20 eliminates the wind from the head and face. Qian zheng is the extra acupoint used for facial paralysis. The location of Qian zheng is 0.5 to 1 cun anterior to the auricular lobe. ST-4, ST-2 and GB-14 are the local points for the facial paralysis. LI-4 is for the facial and head problems. ST-36 and ST-37 are the most important main points. Deep needling is used for ST-36 and ST-37 with the slightly inclined direction to upper body. The depth of needles on ST-36 and

ST-37 have to be 2-3 cun depending on the size of feet. ST-36 and ST-37 regulate the face. The accompanying points are for regulating the local area. ST-44 clears the heat on the stomach channel. Jia cheng jiang is the extra acupoint for the facial paralysis. The location of Jia cheng jiang is 1 cun lateral to CV-24 ( Cheng jiang ). Strong manipulation on the healthy side and soft manipulation on the pathological side are used. The depth of needle has to be shallow. The treatment is applied everyday or once for 2 days.

### <204> Facial spasm

The TCM causes of facial spasm are similar to facial paralysis. Medical consultation is essential. The wind is the main cause of this problem. The main treatment idea is to eliminate the wind and regulate the local area.

The main points : LI-20 ( Ying xiang ), GB-31 ( Feng shi ), ST-44 ( Nei ting ), LI-4 ( He gu ), GB-20 ( Feng chi ), ST-2 ( Si bai ), Liv-2 ( Xing jian ), ST-6 ( Jia che ), LI-3 ( San jian )

The accompanying points : ST-44 ( Nei ting ), Qian zheng ( Ex ), GB-34 ( Yang ling quan ), LI-10 ( Shou san li ), TB-17 ( Yi feng ), Liv-3 ( Tai chong )

To eliminate the wind, calming the liver is necessary. You can refer to the point explanation of facial nerve paralysis. The spasm is a kind of internal wind and clearing the liver heat is added in this prescription. The distant points are important. The strong manipulation is used for the distant points and the soft manipulation is used for the local points.

### <205> Intercostal neuralgia

It can be a kind of inflammation or trauma. Medical consultation is essential. The main TCM treatment idea is to clears the heat and inflammation on the gall bladder channel and remove the Qi stagnation on the gall bladder channel.

The main points : SP-21 ( Da bao ), TB-3 ( Zhong zhu ), GB-41 ( Zu lin qi ), Liv-2 ( Xing jian ), GB-34 ( Yang ling quan ), Ashi points, TB-6 ( Zhi gou ), Liv-13 ( Zhang men )

The accompanying points : SP-9 ( Yin ling quan ), GB-43 ( Xia xi ), TB-5 ( Wai guan ), ST-40 ( Feng long ), PC-4 ( Xi men ), BL-19 ( Dan shu ), BL-18 ( Gan shu )

GB-34 is the most commonly used acupoint to eliminate the pathogen on the gall bladder channel. It removes the damp heat too. TB-6 is the same family channel point with gall bladder channel. SP-21 is the grand luo connecting point to stop pain on the lateral sides. GB-41, Liv-2 and TB-5 regulate the Qi stagnation on the lateral sides. PC-4 connects with liver channel. SP-9 eliminates the dampness. Liv-13 eliminates the intercostal pain. ST-40 eliminates the phlegm that blocks the intercostal region. BL-18 is the back shu point of liver. The strong manipulation is used. Bleeding method using cupping can be used on the ashi points.

### <206> Multiple sclerosis – lower limbs

The symptoms of MS can improve with acupuncture. But for more effective treatment, TCM herbal medicine is necessary. Medical consultation is essential. This is genetic problem and in TCM view, it originates from deficiency of kidneys essence. The organs responsible for this problem are liver, spleen, kidneys and lung. It is related with wind, dampness and deficiency of kidneys. The main treatment idea is to eliminate the wind damp to remove the inflammation, and improve the movement of articulation. Nourishing the kidneys and liver is important.

The main points : BL-40 ( Wei zhong ), Liv-3 ( Tai chong ), SP-4 ( Gong sun ), GB-30 ( Huan tiao ), SP-6 ( San yin jiao ), GB-39 ( Xuan zhong ), ST-36 ( Zu san li ), GB-34 ( Yang ling quan ), PC-6 ( Nei guan

), K-1 ( Yong quan ), Chinese scalp acupuncture ( movement, sense area )

The accompanying points : BL-23 ( Shen shu ), GB-20 ( Feng chi ), Shang ba feng ( Ex ), SI-3 ( Hou xi ), K-7 ( Fu liu ), Ba feng ( Ex ), Liv-2 ( Xing jian ), GV-20 ( Bai hui )

The prescription is the combination of local points and the points that eliminate the wind damp. SP-6 eliminates the dampness but also nourishes kidneys and liver. SP-4 is the luo connecting point of SP channel. K-3 is the Yuan source point of kidneys. Ba feng and Shang ba feng are the extra acupoints. Ba feng are 8 points that are located on each fingers of feet and Shang ba feng on the dorsal sides of feet e about 1 cun above the Ba feng. GB-39 is the hui meeting point of essence and it nourishes the kidneys essence. The medium level manipulation is used. Treatment is done everyday or once for 2 days. Deep needling is necessary. One needle for two points like GB-34 to SP-9 and K-3 to BL-60 is used. Chinese scalp acupuncture is used.

### <207> Multiple sclerosis – upper limbs

The symptoms of MS can improve with acupuncture. But for more effective treatment, TCM herbal medicine is necessary. Medical consultation is essential. This is genetic problem and in TCM view, it originates from deficiency of kidneys essence. The organs responsible for this problem are liver, spleen, kidneys and lung. It is related with wind and dampness, deficiency of kidneys. The main treatment idea is to eliminate the wind damp to remove the inflammation, and improve the movement of articulation. Nourishing the kidneys and liver is important.

The main points : SP-6 ( San yin jiao ), K-1 ( Yong quan ), TB-5 ( Wai guan ), TB-4 ( Yang chi ), Ba xie ( Ex ), LI-4 ( He gu ), Liv-3 ( Tai chong ), LI-11 ( Qu chi ), Chinese scalp acupuncture ( movement, sense area )

The accompanying points : LI-15 ( Jian yu ), SI-3 ( Hou xi ), BL-23 ( Shen shu ), BL-18 ( Gan shu ), SI-6 ( Yang lao ), PC-3 ( Qu ze ), Shang Ba xie ( Ex )

The local points are used to eliminate the damp wind on the local area. The Yang channels are used much because the Yang channels dominate and control the movement of body. Ba xie is the extra acupoint on the feet. Ba xie is at between the fingers and Shang Ba xie is about 1 cun above the Ba xie. The medium level manipulation is used. Treatment is done everyday or once for 2 days. Deep needling is necessary. One needle for two points like LI-11 to Ht-3 and TB-5 to PC-6 is used. Chinese scalp acupuncture is used.

### <208> Myelitis

This disease is the inflammation of spinal cord and the nerve senses can be paralyzed. Medical consultation is essential. In TCM view, the cause is deficiency of Yin or Yang in liver and kidneys essence. The main treatment idea is to control the symptoms like fever or heat, numbness, digestion, urination or constipation and to treat the cause of diseases like tonifying the Yin or Yang, essence, move blood etc. If any other symptoms are known, you can add the treatments for those symptoms.

The main points : GV-8 ( Jin suo ), K-3 ( Tai xi ), PC-6 ( Nei guan ), ST-38 ( Tiao kou ), GV-12 ( Shen zhu ), BL-18 ( Gan shu ), GV-4 ( Ming men ), GV-11 ( Shen dao ), K-1 ( Yong quan ), CV-4 ( Guan yuan )

The accompanying points : GV-20 ( Bai hui ), GV-26 ( Shui gou ), Ht-7 ( Shen men ), BL-25 ( Da chang shu ), BL-23 ( Shen shu ), GB-37 ( Guang ming ), LI-11 ( Qu chi ), SP-4 ( Gong sun ), SP-6 ( San yin jiao )

In case of lower limbs paralysis : GB-39 ( Xuan zhong ), ST-36 ( Zu san li ), ST-40 ( Feng long ), SP-8 ( Di ji ), Liv-3 ( Tai chong ), GB-31 ( Feng shi )

In case of mal functions of urinary bladder or rectum : Lu-5 ( Chi ze ) : reducing method or bloodletting technique, CV-2 ( Qu gu ), SP-9 ( Yin ling quan ), BL-28 ( Pang guang shu ), K-9 ( Zhu bin ), K-7 ( Fu liu ), BL-64 ( Jing gu )

The prescription is comprised of treatment of causes and symptoms. In this prescription, tonifying the Yin, Yang of kidneys and liver is the main treatment method. The accompanying points are for the symptoms. Myelitis needs treatment of TCM herbal medicine to improve the effects of treatment. The strong manipulation is used. Select the points following the symptoms.

### <209> Sciatica

In TCM view, Sciatica is from deficiency of liver and kidneys and pathogens of wind damp on the local area. Medical consultation is essential. The main treatment idea is to eliminate the wind to relieve the pain, eliminate the wind damp and nourish liver and kidneys. The local points and the distant points are used together.

The main points : Zuo gu ( Ex ), GB-34 ( Yang ling quan ), Jia ji ( Ex. L3~L5), BL-31 ( Shang liao ), Ashi, GB-30 ( Huan tiao ), BL-36 ( Cheng fu ), BL-40 ( Wei zhong ), BL-60 ( Kun lun ), GB-41 ( Zu lin qi )

If the pain is perceived more on the BL channel, use the points on the BL channel. If the pain is perceived more on the GB, Liv or SP channel, use the points on the those channels.

The accompanying points : BL-32 ( Ci liao ), GB-39 ( Xuan zhong ), BL-54 ( Zhi bian ), BL-37 ( Yin men ), BL-57 ( Cheng shan )

In case of kidneys deficiency : K-3 ( Tai xi ), SP-6 ( San yin jiao )

In case mental stress aggravates the pain : GV-20 ( Bai hui ), Ht-7 ( Shen men ), PC-6 ( Nei guan )

GB-30 is the essential point for Sciatica. It removes the wind damp on the Sciatic nerve. BL-40 relieves the pain on the back of leg ( BL channel ) and it also moves the blood. BL-31, BL-32, Jia ji and Ashi are the local points for the Sciatica. Jia ji is the extra acupoint. Accompanying points are on the channel where the pains are perceived. Zuo gu is the extra acupoint for the Sciatica. This acupoint is located on the back of the thigh, about 7 cm below the buttock crease, in the depression between the biceps femoris and semitendinosus muscles. This acupoint has a good effect on pain of sciatica. It removes blood stagnation and relieves the pain. Use the long needle for thigh and GB-30. The strong manipulation is used. The electronic acupuncture can be used.

### <210> Trigeminal neuralgia

There can be many causing factors of trigeminal neuralgia. Medical consultation is essential. In TCM view the pain happens when there are the wind damp pathogens, heat, blood stagnation or blockage of phlegm. The main treatment idea is to eliminate the wind damp, heat, blood stagnation, transform the phlegm and relieve the pain. In chronic cases, nourishing the body is necessary.

The main points : Liv-2 ( Xing jian ), ST-2 ( Si bai ), GB-31 ( Feng shi ), BL-2 ( Zan zhu ), ST-7 ( Xia guan ), GB-43 ( Xia xi ), LI-4 ( He gu ), ST-36 ( Zu san li ), GB-14 ( Yang bai ), GB-20 ( Feng chi ), Tai yang ( Ex ) : bloodletting technique

The accompanying points : Liv-3 ( Tai chong ), LI-11 ( Qu chi ), GB-41 ( Zu lin qi ), ST-44 ( Nei ting ), TB-5 ( Wai guan ), LI-3 ( San jian ), Liv-3 ( Tai chong ), K-3 ( Tai xi ), Jia cheng jiang ( Ex )

Tai yang is the extra acupoint to relieve the pain on the lateral side of the face. Jia cheng jiang is the extra acupoint to relieve the pain on the lateral side of the mouth. LI-4 is used to treat the face pain. ST-44 clears the heat on the ST channel that passes the face. GB-20 eliminates the wind from the face and head. K-3 nourishes the kidneys. The light or medium level manipulation is used. The strong manipulation can be used for the severe pain area. The electric acupuncture can be used for this problem.

# | 21 |

# Pediatric health issues

### <211> Infantile nearsightedness ( Myopia )

The infant's nerves and tendon system are not fixed yet because it is still on the process of growing. Medical consultation is essential. The cause of infantile nearsightedness can be from watching TV, playing game too much, or cel phone etc. For the mental and emotional health of children, too much TV or games are not recommended. The main treatment idea in acupuncture is to activate the Qi and blood on eyes and to nourish the liver and kidneys.

The main points : GB-37 ( Guang ming ), Yi ming ( Ex ), GB-20 ( Feng chi ), BL-1 ( Jing ming ) : you must follow the safety guide of needle technique, ST-1 ( Cheng qi ), Liv-3 ( Tai chong ), K-7 ( Fu liu )
The accompanying points : SI-3 ( Hou xi ), ST-36 ( Zu san li ), Liv-8 ( Qu quan ), GB-16 ( Mu chuang ), BL-10 ( Tian zhu ), GB-43 ( Xia xi ), TB-3 ( Zhong zhu )

The prescription is comprised of local acupoints and the points that nourish kidneys and liver. Some special points for the eyesight are used like K-7, GB-43, GB-16 and GB-37. The GB channels are used much because GB and liver channel is closely related with eyesight. The medium level manipulation is used. Stop reading books or watching TV during the period of treatment.

### <212> Pediatric acute seizure

This happens with high fever or meningitis. Medical consultation is essential. The main treatment idea in acupuncture is to clear the internal heat and eliminate the internal or external wind. TCM herbal medicine for this case will help a lot. The high fever can be dangerous for a baby.

The main points : GV-1 ( Chang qiang ), GV-26 ( Shui gou ), GV-20 ( Bai hui ), GV-12 ( Shen zhu ), LI-4 ( He gu ), K-1 ( Yong quan ) : pressing with finger

In case of high fever : Bloodletting technique on Er jian ( the point of ear tips in auricular acupuncture )

The accompanying points : K-10 ( Yin gu ), LI-1 ( Shang yang ) or other Jing well points of hands, Ashi on the back and abdominal area.

In case of acute seizure, it is not easy to do acupuncture. It is good to consider bloodletting technique. Treatment using GV channel is essential to clear the high fever. GV-12 is used for seizure and it also nourishes the body. GV-20 is to eliminate the wind and control the body balance. GV-1 is the essential point for infantile seizure. K-10 nourishes the kidneys Yin to hold the uprising wind. LI-4 clears the heat in the head. GV-26 awakens the consciousness to make the mind clear. Moxibustion is used on GV-12, GV-20 and GV-1. Bleeding method is used on LI-1. Other points are needled. Ring press needles are used on the ashi on the back and the abdominal area.

### <213> Pediatric asthma

This problem can happen with many causes like allergy, inborn constitution or immunity. Medical consultation is essential. Usually the babies have weak spleen and excess liver syndromes. Balancing the soil and wood elements, treating the respiratory system is essential.

The main points : PC-6 ( Nei guan ) : In case the localization is not clear because of too young age, you can omit this point, BL-12 ( Feng men ), CV-17 ( Shan zhong ), GV-12 ( Shen zhu ), GV-10 ( Ling tai ), Ding chuan ( Ex ), LI-10 ( Shou san li )

The accompanying points : ST-36 ( Zu san li ), CV-12 ( Zhong wan ), Lu-5 ( Chi ze ), Liv-2 ( Xing jian ), Area on the neck, shoulder, chest and the back : it is good to use acupuncture or massage by finger.

GV-12 and GV-10 are used a lot for pediatric problems. It nourishes body and also clears the pathologic heat as well. BL-12 expels the external wind that causes the asthma. Ding chuan is the extra acupoint for asthma or respiratory problems. The location is on the back, 0.5 cun lateral to the lower border of the spinous process of the 7th cervical vertebra. Treatment of spleen is essential for asthma because spleen nourishes lung. In case of infantile, moxibustion is used on GV-12 and GV-10 and magnets are used on other main points and ring press needles are used on the accompanying points. In case of adolescents, moxibustion is used on GV-12 and GV-10, and needles are used for other main points and ring press needles are used on the accompanying points.

### <214> Pediatric constitutional weakness

Constitutional weakness can continue for whole life if not treated properly in childhood. Medical consultation is essential. The main causes are insufficient nutrients when the mother was pregnant or in the childhood or genetically weak. Usually the spleen and stomach or kidneys is in deficiency. The main treatment idea is to activate the lung, to tonify spleen and kidneys or Qi and blood.

The main points : ST-36 ( Zu san li ), BL-23 ( Shen shu ), GV-12 ( Shen zhu ), GV-4 ( Ming men ), GB-25 ( Jing men ), CV-4 ( Guan yuan )

# ACUPUNCTURE PROTOCOLS FOR 300 HEALTH CONDITIONS - 193

The accompanying points : GV-9 ( Zhi yang ), SP-10 ( Xue hai ), SP-6 ( San yin jiao ), CV-12 ( Zhong wan ), TB-2 ( Ye men ), Lu-6 ( Kong zui ), BL-17 ( Ge shu ), BL-12 ( Feng men )

It is not necessary to use all these points. You can choose some from your own diagnosis. GB-25 is the front mu point of kidneys to tonify kidneys. The points are to tonify kidneys and spleen. BL-17 is to nourish the blood. Lu-6 is the Xi cleft point of lung to activate the lung. BL-12 eliminates the external wind that easily causes the inflammation for low immunity persons ( weakness ). The other points are to tonify the body or Yin and Yang. Moxibustion is used on the main points for 3~5 times for one session. Select some accompanying points to needle with soft manipulation. Use less number of needles.

### <215> Pediatric diarrhea

Pediatric diarrhea is mainly from deficiency of spleen if not has infection. Medical consultation is essential. The main treatment idea is to regulate the digestion system through spleen, stomach and large intestine.

The main points : ST-36 ( Zu san li ), LI-11 ( Qu chi ), ST-34 ( Liang qiu ), SP-9 ( Yin ling quan ), ST-25 ( Tian shu ), Zhi xie ( Ex ), Si feng ( Ex )

The accompanying points : For fever : LI-4 ( He gu ), GV-14 ( Da zhui )

For vomiting : PC-6 ( Nei guan )

ST-25 is the front mu point of large intestine. Zhi xie is the extra acupoint for diarrhea. The location is 2.5 cun below the belly button on the CV channel. ST-34 is the Xi cleft point of stomach channel. Si feng is the extra acupoint to treat the digestion problems of babies. The location is on the palmar surface, in the midpoint of the transverse creases of the proximal interphalangeal joints of the index, middle, ring and little fingers. If the baby has the fever or vomiting, you can use the accompanying points. Use the gross angle needle on Si feng to squeeze out the yellow and white fatty materials. The medium level needling manipulation is used on other points. If the infantile does not want to be needled, the ring press needles are used on Si feng and magnets are used on other points.

### <216> Pediatric febrile convulsion

The internal or external causes can make fever for babies. If the fever is high it causes convulsion. Medical consultation is essential. The main treatment idea is to clear the heat and calm the wind. The organs or channel related with this problem are liver, pericardium, kidneys and GV channel.

The main points : Shi xuan ( Ex ) : bloodletting technique, Feng guan ( Ex ), Yin tang ( Ex ), Tai yang ( Ex ) : possibly do bloodletting technique, GB-31 ( Feng shi ), LI-11 ( Qu chi ), LI-4 ( He gu ), GV-14 ( Da zhui ), PC-8 ( Lao gong )

The accompanying points : GV-20 ( Bai hui ), GV-12 ( Shen zhu ), Er jian ( the point of ear tips of auricular acupuncture ) : bloodletting technique, K-1 ( Yong quan ), TB-5 ( Wai guan )

Yin tang and Tai yang are the extra acupoints to eliminate the heat from the head. Feng guan is the extra acupoint for febrile convulsion. The metacarpophalangeal joint of the index finger is called Feng guan. Shi xuan is the extra acupoint for the emergency situation. The location is on the ends of the fingers. GV channels are used to clear the internal high fever and to calm the convulsion. LI-11 and LI-4 clears the heat. PC-8 clears the heat from pericardium to open the orifices. TB-5 eliminates the external pathogen or wind. K-1 opens the orifices and awakens the mind. The bleeding method is used on Shi xuan and Feng guan. The strong needling manipulation is used on other points.

### <217> Pediatric functional dyspepsia ( difficulty in digestion )

Dyspepsia is about difficulty in digestion. Medical consultation is essential. The main treatment idea is to regulate the digestive system like stomach, spleen and liver.

The main points : Liv-3 ( Tai chong ), Si feng ( Ex ), ST-36 ( Zu san li ), Yin tang ( Ex )
The accompanying points : ST-37 ( Shang ju xu ), LI-4 ( He gu ), PC-6 ( Nei guan )
In case of nervousness : Ht-7 ( Shen men ), GV-20 ( Bai hui )

Si feng is the extra acupoint for infantile dyspepsia. The location is on the palmar surface, in the midpoint of the transverse creases of the proximal interphalangeal joints of the index, middle, ring and little fingers. ST-36 and CV-12 regulate the digestion. LI-4 and ST-25 regulate the function of large intestine. Yin tang is the extra acupoint to calm the mind. Ht-7 and liv-3 calm the mind. Use the gross angle needle to squeeze out the yellow and white fatty materials from Si feng. Soft needling manipulation is used on other points and remove the needles immediately after the manipulation. Used tonifying methods.

### <218> Pediatric night astonishment

Astonishment is usually about kidneys, liver and gall bladder. Medical consultation is essential. But in acupuncture treatment we focus on the GV channel to clear the mind. Treating on GV channel can include the treatment on kidneys, liver and gall bladder.

The main points : Liv-2 ( Xing jian ), Ht-7 ( Shen men ), GB-43 ( Xia xi ), LI-2 ( Er jian ), GV-12 ( Shen zhu ), GV-4 ( Ming men )
The accompanying points : ST-36 ( Zu san li ), Both sides of the vertebrae, all area of abdomen, area of fontanelle : good to use massage technique or seven stars needles

GV-12 awakens the mind and calms the astonishment of baby. GV-4 tonifies the kidneys yang. LI-2 calms the astonishment. The sides of vertebrae, all area of abdomen and area of fontanelle calm the mind and the movement of Qi. Moxibustion is used on the main points. Use the seven stars needles softly on the accompanying points

### <219> Pediatric non febrile convulsion

Medical consultation is essential. The main cause is internal wind that is generated from liver and gall bladder and that is related with GV channel, tendons and muscles. The main treatment idea is to eliminate the wind and regulate the GV channel, calm the tendons and muscles.

The main points : GB-31 ( Feng shi ), GV-14 ( Da zhui ), SI-3 ( Hou xi ), GV-8 ( Jin suo ), Liv-3 ( Tai chong ), GV-26 ( Shui gou )

The accompanying points : PC-6 ( Nei guan ), GV-12 ( Shen zhu ), Liv-2 ( Xing jian ), GB-34 ( Yang ling quan ), LI-4 ( He gu ), GB-43 ( Xia xi ), An mian ( Ex )

GV-14 clears the heat from the all Yang channel to calm the convulsion. GB-8 relaxes the tendons. SI-3 opens GV channel to calm the convulsion. GB-34 relaxes the muscles and tendons. GV-12 calms the convulsion. An mian is the extra acupoint to treat insomnia but here it can be used to eliminate the wind from the head. The location of An mian is the midpoint between TB-17 ( Yi feng ) and GB-20 ( Feng chi ). Liv-3 calms the internal wind from liver. GV-26 awakens the mind. The strong needling manipulation is used to calm the wind. Remove the needles immediately after the manipulation.

### <220> Pediatric stomatitis

Stomatitis is inflamed and sore mouth. In case of pediatric stomatitis, it is closely related with mal nutrition, deficiency of spleen and stomach or liver excess. Medical consultation is essential. The main treatment idea is to tonify the spleen and stomach. If any other cause is known, you can add the treatment.

The main points : ST-36 ( Zu san li ), Liv-3 ( Tai chong ), GV-4 ( Ming men ), LI-10 ( Shou san li ), BL-20 ( Pi shu ), GV-12 ( Shen zhu )

The accompanying points : GV-20 ( Bai hui ), You can use seven stars needles on the area on the nape, the Lu channel and the frontal neck, the LI channel on the upper limbs, the BL channel on the back, the ST channel on the leg,

GV-12 nourishes the body. BL-20 and LI-10 tonify the spleen. GV-4 increases the kidneys yang to warm the spleen and stomach. The accompanying points are to increase the effect of treatment. You can use the seven stars needle or the ring press needles. The moxibustion is used 3~5 times for a session.

### <221> Pediatric vomiting

The pediatric vomiting easily happens with deficiency of spleen and stomach or liver excess. Medical consultation is essential. The main treatment idea is to tonify the spleen and stomach and regulate the digestion.

The main points : Liv-3 ( Tai chong ), Si feng ( Ex ), GV-12 ( Shen zhu ), ST-36 ( Zu san li ), GV-4 ( Ming men )

The accompanying points : PC-6 ( Nei guan ), Seven stars needling on the area of the ST channel on the abdomen, BL channel on the back, CV channel, Lu channel, ST, SP channel on the legs or LI channel on upper limbs.

GV-12 nourishes the body and stops vomiting. GV-4 increases the kidneys Yang to warm the spleen and stomach. Si feng treats the mal nutrition of babies and treats the pediatric vomiting. Moxibustion is used on GV-12 and GV-4 for 3~5 times a session. Ring press needles are used on Si feng and the accompanying points.

### <222> Poliomyelitis ( initial stage ) – abdominal muscles

Poliomyelitis is an infectious disease caused by the poliovirus. Medical consultation is essential. The main treatment idea is to regulate the local area with needling.

The main points : ST-25 ( Tian shu ), CV-9 ( Shui fen ), CV-4 ( Guan yuan ), SP-21 ( Da bao ), Jia ji ( Ex, corresponding points ), GB-41 ( Dai mai )

The accompanying points : CV-10 ( Xia wan ), Liv-13 ( Zhang men ), CV-12 ( Zhong wan ), ST-21 ( Liang men ), GB-25 ( Jing men )

Jia ji is the extra acupoint to eliminate the local paralysis, pain or Bi syndrome etc. CV-4 is to tonify the Qi and blood to increase the protection of body from pathogen. SP-21 is the grand luo connecting point on the thorax. In the initial stage, basically many points are needled superficially with soft manipulation. In the chronic stage, the points are needled deeply with strong manipulation. The pathological side are needled mainly.

### <223> Poliomyelitis ( initial stage ) – lower limbs

Poliomyelitis is an infectious disease caused by the poliovirus. Medical consultation is essential. The main treatment idea is to regulate the local area with needling.

The main points : ST-36 ( Zu san li ), SP-6 ( San yin jiao ), GB-34 ( Yang ling quan ), BL-37 ( Yin men ), GB-30 ( Huan tiao ), SP-10 ( Xue hai ), K-1 ( Yong quan ), Jian xi ( Ex ), ST-32 ( Fu tu ), Zuo gu ( Ex ), Liv-3 ( Tai chong ), SP-9 ( Yin ling quan )

The accompanying points : GB-40 ( Qiu xu ), GB-31 ( Feng shi ), GV-4 ( Ming men ), BL-32 ( Ci liao ), GV-3 ( Yao yang guan ), other points on the legs.

The points are to regulate the local area and tonify the Qi and blood to increase the protection from the pathogens. GB-34 is the hui meeting point of the tendon. ST-36 tonifies the Qi and also eliminates the dampness. GV-4 increases the kidneys yang to increase the protection from the pathogens. GV-3 warms the body also relieve the lumbar pain. Zuo gu is the extra acupoint for the Sciatica or Bi syndrome on the local area. This acupoint is located on the back of the thigh, about 7 cm below the buttock crease, in the depression between the biceps femoris and semitendinosus muscles. This acupoint has a good effect on pain of sciatica or local area. It removes blood stagnation and relieves the pain. Jian xi is the extra acupoint to strengthen the knee. This extra point is located 3 cun directly above the center point of the superior border of the patella. In the initial stage, basically many points are needled superficially with soft manipulation. In the chronic stage, the points are needled deeply with strong manipulation. The pathological side are needled mainly.

### <224> Poliomyelitis ( initial stage ) – neck

Poliomyelitis is an infectious disease caused by the poliovirus. Medical consultation is essential. The main treatment idea is to regulate the local area with needling.

The main points : SI-3 ( Hou xi ), TB-16 ( Tian you ), BL-40 ( Wei zhong ) : bloodletting technique, ST-9 ( Ren ying ), LI-17 ( Tian ding ), Jia ji ( Ex, corresponding to C2~C6 ), GB-20 ( Feng chi ), BL-10 ( Tian zhu ), GV-15 ( Ya men )

The accompanying points : BL-64 ( Jing gu ), BL-65 ( Shu gu ), TB-17 ( Tian rong ), GB-12 ( Wan gu ), GV-16 ( Feng fu )

Jia ji is the extra acupoint to treat the local Bi syndrome or pain. In the initial stage, basically many points are needled superficially with soft manipulation. In the chronic stage, the points are needled deeply with strong manipulation. The pathological side are needled mainly.

### <225> Poliomyelitis ( initial stage ) – upper limbs

Poliomyelitis is an infectious disease caused by the poliovirus. Medical consultation is essential. The main treatment idea is to regulate the local area with needling.

The main points : TB-6 ( Zhi gou ), LI-15 ( Jian yu ), Jia ji ( Ex. Corresponding to C5~C7, T1 ), Lu-5 ( Chi ze ), Jing bi ( Ex ), TB-14 ( Jian liao ), SI-8 ( Xiao hai ), LI-4 ( He gu ), SP-6 ( San yin jiao )

The accompanying points : TB-9 ( Si du ), Ht-1 ( Ji quan ), GV-14 ( Da zhui ), SI-3 ( Hou xi ), SI-7 ( Zhi zheng ), LI-11 ( Qu chi ), TB-5 ( Wan guan )

Jing bi is the extra acupoint to eliminate the local pain or Bi syndrome. Jing bi is located 1 cun directly superior to the point between the medial 1/3 and lateral 2/3 of the clavicle. Jia ji is the extra acupoint to eliminate the local Bi syndrome or pain. In the initial stage, basically many points are needled superficially with soft manipulation. In the chronic stage, the points are needled deeply with strong manipulation. The pathological side are needled mainly.

### <226> Poliomyelitis ( initial stage ) – facial muscles

Poliomyelitis is an infectious disease caused by the poliovirus. Medical consultation is essential. The main treatment idea is to regulate the local area with needling.

The main points : GB-34 ( Yang ling quan ), ST-36 ( Zu san li ), Qian zheng ( Ex ), ST-6 ( Jia che ), ST-44 ( Nei ting ), TB-17 ( Yi feng ), LI-4 ( He gu ), LI-11 ( Qu chi )

The accompanying points : ST-37 ( Shang ju xu ), ST-40 ( Feng long ), ST-7 ( Xia guan ), Yin tang ( Ex ), CV-24 ( Cheng jiang ), GB-2 ( Ting hui ), ST-4 ( Di cang ), Jia cheng jiang ( Ex )

The point prescription is similar to those of facial paralysis. Mainly use the channels that pass the face. Qian zheng is the extra acupoint to treat the facial paralysis. The location is 0.5-1.0 cun anterior to the earlobe. Jia cheng jiang is the extra acupoint to treat facial paralysis. The location is 1 cun lateral to CV-24 ( Cheng jiang ). In the initial stage, basically many points are needled superficially with soft manipulation. In the chronic stage, the points are needled deeply with strong manipulation. The pathological side are needled mainly.

# | 22 |

# Respiratory system

### <227> Bronchial asthma

The main organs responsible for asthma are lung, kidneys and spleen. Medical consultation is essential. And sometimes excess of liver is related. All asthma has the pathogen of phlegm and treatment of phlegm is necessary. The prescription is comprised of treatment of activating the lung, tonifying kidneys and spleen and transforming the phlegm.

The main points : PC-6 ( Nei guan ), K-27 ( Shu fu ), ST-40 ( Feng long ), Ding chuan ( Ex ), CV-22 ( Tian tu ), CV-17 ( Shan zhong ), Lu-7 ( Lie que ), K-6 ( Zhao hai )

The accompanying points : CV-12 ( Zhong wan ), LI-4 ( He gu ), K-7 ( Fu liu ), SP-4 ( Gong sun ), GV-14 ( Da zhui ), Lu-5 ( Chi ze )

For chronic case, CV-6 ( Qi hai ), BL-13 ( Fei shu ), ST-36 ( Zu san li )

For lung heat : Lu-10 ( Yu ji )

Ding chuan is the extra acupoint for asthma. The location is 0.5 cun lateral to GV-14 ( Da zhui ). CV-22 transforms the phlegm and make the Qi go down to calm the asthma. K-27 regulates the respiration. CV-17 opens the chest. BL-13 is the back shu point of lung and it nourishes the lung. Lu-5 reduces the lung excess. LI-4 clears the heat in the lung. CV-4 tonifies the lower burner like kidneys. ST-36 strengthens the spleen and also eliminates the phlegm. ST-40 transforms the phlegm. CV-12 transforms the phlegm and regulates the middle burner. The strong manipulation is used. The needle is removed immediately after needling to the four directions is used on CV-17.

### <228> Bronchiectasis

Bronchiectasis happens when the airway is damaged. Medical consultation is essential. The symptoms can be infection, pneumonia, asthma etc. The treatment has to be done with medications. The main treatment idea is to activate the lung, eliminate the infection and to relieve the symptoms.

The main points : Lu-7 ( Lie que ), K-6 ( Zhao hai ), Ding chuan ( Ex ), Lu-5 ( Chi ze ), ST-36 ( Zu san li ), LI-4 ( He gu ), CV-22 ( Tian tu ), BL-13 ( Fei shu ), ST-40 ( Feng long )

The accompanying points : K-7 ( Fu liu ), BL-43 ( Gao huang ), GV-12 ( Shen zhu ), BL-12 ( Feng men ), CV-17 ( Shan zhong ), Lu-6 ( Kong zui )

LI-4 clears the heat in the superior burner, the lung. BL-13 activates and nourishes the lung. Ding chuan is the extra acupoint for difficulty in respiration. The location of Ding chuan is 0.5 cun lateral to GV-14 ( Da zhui ). BL-12 opens lung and eliminates the external pathogen in lung. CV-22 transforms the phlegm and makes the Qi descend to calm the asthma. BL-43 nourishes the lung. Lu-5 reduces the pathogen in the lung. Lu-6 activates and regulates the lung. ST-40 transforms the phlegm. CV-17 opens the chest. GV-12 nourishes the body and stops asthma and cough. The strong needling manipulation is used. The moxibustion is used for the chronic cases.

### <229> Bronchitis

Bronchitis is an inflammation of the lining of bronchial tubes. Medical consultation is essential. The patient will cough up thickened mucus. It can be either chronic or acute. The main treatment idea is to activate the lung, eliminate the phlegm and depending on the syndromes, the cooling the lung heat method can be used.

The main points : Lu-7 ( Lie que ), K-6 ( Zhao hai ), Ding chuan ( Ex ), BL-13 ( Fei shu ), CV-22 ( Tian tu ), ST-40 ( Feng long ) : bloodletting technique

The accompanying points : Lu-5 ( Chi ze ), K-7 ( Fu liu ), BL-12 ( Feng men ), SP-4 ( Gong sun ), LI-4 ( He gu ), CV-17 ( Shan zhong ), Lu-6 ( Kong zui )

LI-4 clears the lung heat and eliminates the external pathogen. BL-13 activates the lung. Ding chuan is the extra acupoint to treat the asthma or difficulty in respiration. BL-12 eliminates the external pathogen from lung. CV-22 transforms the phlegm and makes the Qi descend to calm the cough. Lu-5 reduces the pathogens in lung. Lu-6 activates the lung function. ST-40 transforms the phlegm. CV-17 opens the lung to relieve the chest pain. The strong manipulation is used for the acute case. In case of chronic case, soft manipulation is used.

### <230> Cardiac asthma

This problem can happen with the left heart failure. Medical consultation is essential. The liquid can accumulate in the lung and build the pulmonary edema. The patient can experience coughing or wheezing. If the pulmonary edema happens, that is the emergency situation. The main treatment idea is to activate and regulate the function of heat and lung and eliminate the accumulation of liquid in the lung.

The main points : SI-1 ( Shao ze ), K-7 ( Fu liu ), PC-4 ( Xi men ), Lu-6 ( Kong zui ), K-27 ( Shu fu ), BL-15 ( Xin shu ), Ht-3 ( Shao hai ), GV-22 ( Xin hui ), Ht-8 ( Shao fu ), Lu-1 ( Zhong fu )

The accompanying points : ST-40 ( Feng long ) : bloodletting technique, Du yin ( Ex ) : bloodletting technique, GV-10 ( Ling tai ), GV-20 ( Bai hui ), Ding chuan ( Ex ), SP-4 ( Gong sun ), GV-12 ( Shen zhu ), BL-12 ( Feng men ), BL-13 ( Fei shu )

Acute outbreak : PC-6 ( Nei guan ), GV-26 ( Shui gou )

It is not necessary to use all these acupoints. It is better use less number of acupoints because this patient is probably in deficiency situation. Just choose the proper acupoints following your own diagnosis result. PC-4 is the Xi cleft point of pericardium and it regulates the heart. Xi cleft point is used for the emergency situation. Ht-3 is the He sea point of heart channel and it regulates the heart functions. SI-1 is the Jing well point of small intestine and used for the emergency situation. BL-15 is the back shu point of heart and it nourishes and activates the heart. GV-10 activates the heart. GV-20 tonifies the Qi. GV-22 opens the orifice to clear the mind and awareness. Lu-1 is the front mu point of lung and it regulates and recuperates the lung function. K-27 regulates the respiration. Ding chuan relieve the difficulty in respiration. Ding chuan is the extra acupoint to relieve the difficulty in respiration. The location of Ding chuan is 0.5 cun lateral to GV-14 ( Da zhui ). In emergency and acute case GV-26 is used to open the orifice. The bleeding method is used on the SI-1. The medium level manipulation is used. In case of acute case, GV-26 ( Shui gou ) can be used.

### <231> Cough

Cough has many different causes but the cough itself is the symptom of mal function of lung. Medical consultation is essential. If any cause is known, it is necessary to treat that cause. Here the prescription is for treating the symptom, cough. The main treatment idea is to eliminate the blockage of lung, eliminate the phlegm and recover the function of lung. The organs related with cough are lung, kidneys, spleen and liver. But in this prescription we focus on the treatment of lung.

The main points : Lu-5 ( Chi ze ), CV-22 ( Tian tu ), CV-12 ( Zhong wan ), BL-13 ( Fei shu ), BL-43 ( Gao huang ), Lu-7 ( Lie que ), K-6 ( Zhao hai )
The accompanying points : K-27 ( Shu fu ), SP-6 ( San yin jiao ), Lu-1 ( Zhong fu ), CV-14 ( Ju que ), GB-20 ( Feng chi ), K-7 ( Fu liu ), BL-23 ( Shen shu ), GB-21 ( Jian jing ), CV-17 ( Shan zhong ),
In case of mental stress : Ht-7 ( Shen men ), Liv-3 ( Tai chong ), VG-20 ( Bai hui )

BL-43 nourishes the lung and activates the lung. GV-21 regulates the Qi on the superior burner. Lu-5 reduces the pathogen in the lung. BL-13 regulates the lung. GB-20 eliminates the external wind that was blocking the lung. Lu-1 is the front mu point of lung and it regulates the function of lung. CV-14 is the front mu point of heart and it removes the blockage on the chest and helps the lung function. CV-12 transforms the phlegm and regulates the movement of Qi. The lung channel begins from CV-12, so CV-12 has the function of regulating the lung. K-27 regulates the lung movement. CV-17 opens the chest and relieve the chest pain. CV-22 transforms the phlegm and makes the lung Qi descend to calm the cough. Strong manipulation is used for acute case and soft manipulation is used for chronic case.

### <232> Difficulty in breathing

There are many causes of difficulty in breathing. Medical consultation is essential. Problems can be in the lung or respiratory system, heart, kidneys, stress or liver etc. If any cause is known it is necessary to treat the cause at the same time. In this prescription the main treatment is focused on lung and kidneys. the additional treatment can be used.

The main points : PC-6 ( Nei guan ), SP-4 ( Gong sun ), K-26 ( Yu zhong ), Lu-5 ( Chi ze ), BL-11 ( Da zhu ), BL-13 ( Fei shu ), BL-23 ( Shen shu ), Lu-7 ( Lie que ), K-6 ( Zhao hai ), CV-17 ( Shan zhong )

The accompanying points : BL-42 ( Po hu ), K-7 ( Fu liu ), ST-36 ( Zu san li ), LI-18 ( Fu tu ), ST-9 ( Ren ying )

In case of phlegm at the respiratory problem : ST-40 ( Feng long ), CV-22 ( Tian tu ), CV-12 ( Zhong wan ), Lu-1 ( Zhong fu )

In case of heart problem : PC-3 ( Qu ze ), Ht-7 ( Shen men )

In case of hysteria : Liv-3 ( Tai chong ), GV-20 ( Bai hui ), BL-18 ( Gan shu ), GB-34 ( Yang ling quan ), GB-20 ( Feng chi )

Lu-5 reduces the pathogen in the lung. Lu-7 opens the CV channel and lung channel to activate the function. K-26 helps respiration. BL-11 nourishes Yin of lung and essence of kidneys. BL-13 nourishes the lung and regulates the function of lung. CV-17 opens the chest to help respiration. BL-42 nourishes the lung and regulates the corporeal spirit of lung ( po ). Depending on the cases and causes, the accompanying points can be added.

The strong manipulation is used for acute case and the soft manipulation is used for chronic case.

### <233> Emphysema

Emphysema is the lung disease that results from damage to the walls of the alveoli in the lungs. Medical consultation is essential. This can trap the air in the lung and the chest can appear fuller or barrel chested appearance. The main treatment idea is to nourish the lung and recover the function of lung.

The main points : ST-19 ( Bu rong ), LI-10 ( Shou san li ), CV-17 ( Shan zhong ), BL-17 ( Ge shu ), ST-36 ( Zu san li ), Lu-9 ( Tai yuan ), Lu-7 ( Lie que ), K-3 ( Tai xi )

The accompanying points : Lu-1 ( Zhong fu ), CV-4 ( Guan yuan ), K-9 ( Zhu bin ), Lu-5 ( Chi ze ), Liv-3 ( Tai chong )

BL-13 and BL-43 nourish the lung to recover from emphysema rapidly. BL-17 regulates the blood movement. Lu-1 is the front mu point of lung and it regulates the lung functions. ST-19 helps respiration. Lu-5 eliminates the stagnation in the lung. LI-10 strengthens the spleen Qi to recover from the damage rapidly. K-3 is the Yuan source point of kidneys and tonifies the kidneys to nourish the lung. Lu-9 is the Yuan source point of lung and it tonifies the lung. CV-17 will open the chest blockage. K-9 nourishes the kidneys. The strong manipulation is used for acute case. The moxibustion is used for chronic case.

### <234> Pertussis ( Whooping cough, 100 days cough )

This is a highly contagious bacterial disease. Medical consultation is essential. The patients cough so hard that they vomit, break ribs, or become very tired. Children less than one year old have little or no cough and but they have periods where they cannot breathe. In TCM view this is lung heat with phlegm. The main treatment idea is to eliminate the pathogen and detoxify the lung and transform the phlegm. Depending on the different syndromes and patterns the treatment way can be different.

The main points : LI-4 ( He gu ), ST-40 ( Feng long ), PC-6 ( Nei guan ), CV-22 ( Tian tu ), Si feng ( Ex ), Ding chuan ( Ex ), Lu-7 ( Lie que ), K-6 ( Zhao hai )

The accompanying points : GV-12 ( Shen zhu ), K-3 ( Tai xi ), CV-4 ( Guan yuan ), GV-14 ( Da zhui ), BL-23 ( Shen shu )

Si feng is the extra acupoint used for the pediatric cases, especially for the emergency cases. The location is on the palmar surface, in the midpoint of the transverse creases of the proximal interphalangeal joints of the index, middle, ring and little fingers and there are total 8 points on both sides. It treats the whooping cough for children. PC-6 relieves the chest pain and clears the heat on the chest and also transforms the phlegm and calm the cough. LI-4 clears the lung heat and eliminates the pathogen and detoxifies the lung. CV-22 transforms the phlegm and make the Qi descend to calm the coughing. GV-14 clears the body heat. GV-12 stops coughing. ST-40 transforms the phlegm. Ding chuan is the extra acupoint for asthma and difficulty in breathing. The location is 0.5 cun lateral to GV-14 ( Da zhui ). Blood-letting technique is used on Si feng, superficial needling is used on CV-22. Strong manipulation is used.

### <235> Pneumonia

Pneumonia is the inflammation of lung. Medical consultation is essential. There are acute and chronic cases. In case of chronic cases, it is necessary to tonify and nourish the lung, Qi and kidneys. In this prescription, we focus on the acute case only. Acute case is the excess syndrome ( pattern ) in TCM view. The main treatment idea is to clear the lung heat, detoxify the toxin and eliminate the external pathogen.

Moxibustion on BL-13 ( Fei shu ), BL-12 ( Feng men ), ST-36 ( Zu san li ), GV-12 ( Shen zhu ), SI-3 ( Hou xi )

After the symptoms like fever, difficulty in breathing disappear, Moxibustions are used on Lu-5 ( Chi ze ), Lu-1 ( Zhong fu ), GV-4 ( Ming men ), GV-10 ( Ling tai )

Needles on K-3 ( Tai xi ), Lu-10 ( Yu ji ), Lu-7 ( Lie que )

Moxibustion on SI-3 is for the febrile diseases. GV-12 treats the lung problem. GB-20 eliminates the wind from the head. BL-12 eliminates the wind. GV-10 stops coughing. Lu-5 reduces the pathogen in the lung. Lu-1 regulates the lung function to stop coughing. Moxibustion 25 times on SI-3. 3 times on other points.

### <236> Pulmonary tuberculosis

The main treatment idea of pulmonary tuberculosis is to nourish the Yin of lung and eliminate the pathogen from the lung. Medical consultation is essential. There can be many other different syndrome patterns but this is the basic idea of the treatment.

The main points : BL-43 ( Gao huang ) : moxibustion, BL-12 ( Feng men ), Lu-7 ( Lie que ), K-6 ( Zhao hai ), BL-13 ( Fei shu ) : moxibustion, GV-12 ( Shen zhu ), CV-17 ( Shan zhong ), BL-42 ( Po hu ), BL-23 ( Shen shu )

The accompanying points : CV-12 ( Zhong wan ), ST-40 ( Feng long ), ST-36 ( Zu san li ), GV-10 ( Ling tai ), K-3 ( Tai xi ), Lu-10 ( Yu ji ), Lu-5 ( Chi ze ), BL-11 ( Da zhu )

BL-13 and GV-12 nourishes the lung. BL-43 nourishes the Yin of lung. BL-12 eliminates the wind from the lung. Lu-7 is the luo connecting point of lung and it regulates the functions of lung. ST-36 tonifies the Qi of spleen and stomach and increases the lung Qi. BL-11 increases the kidneys essence to nourish the lung. GV-10 stops coughing. CV-12 is the starting point of lung channel and it transforms the phlegm and regulates the middle burner to help the lung recover. Lu-5 reduces the pathogen from the lung. CV-17 opens the chest and relieves the chest pain. BL-42 nourishes the lung and the corporeal spirit of lung. Moxibustion is used for more than 5 times each. Everyday practicing is important.

# | 23 |

# Articulation, Bi syndrome, Muscle weakness etc

### <237> Achilles tendinitis

The main treatment idea is to eliminate the local stagnation of blood and Qi. Medical consultation is essential. The local points are used the most. Tendinitis is closely related with wind damp pathogens and the spleen, liver and gall bladder channels. It is necessary to eliminate the wind damp from the channels.

The main points : BL-60 ( Kun lun ), ST-36 ( Zu san li ), BL-57 ( Cheng shan ) : bloodletting technique, K-5 ( Shui quan ), SP-9 ( Yin ling quan ), K-7 ( Fu liu ), GB-34 ( Yang ling quan ),

The accompanying points : BL-61 ( Pu can ), BL-59 ( Fu yang ), K-3 ( Tai xi ), BL-40 ( Wei zhong ) : bloodletting technique, Ashi, Acupoints on the wrist ( considering the channels of same family with the pain points ).

The local points are used. BL-40 and BL-57 eliminates the blood stagnation. GB-34 eliminates the dampness on the tendons and relieves the pain on the tendons. The wrist corresponds to the ankle and you can choose the acupoints on the wrists. If the pain on the ankle is on the channel of BL, you can choose the acupoint on the channel of SI of the wrist like SI-5, SI-6 or SI-7. If the pain is on the K channel, you can choose the acupoint on the channel of Ht of the wrist like Ht-7 or Ht-6. Strong manipulation is used on the acute case.

### <238> Acute backpain(1)

There are many different kinds of causes of backpain. Medical consultation is essential. Here in this prescription, we only focus on the pain itself. The GV channel, kidneys and BL channel are the most responsible for the back pain. The local and the distant acupoints are used. It is good to use moving body method when you treat the pain of local area. After needling the distant point, let the patient move the local area of problem.

The main points : BL-40 ( Wei zhong ):bloodletting technique, BL-60 ( Kun lun ), Ashi, GV-26 ( Shui gou ), K-2 ( Ran gu ), GB-34 ( Yang ling quan ), Yao tong xue ( Ex )
The accompanying points : GV-20 ( Bai hui ), Liv-3 ( Tai chong ), GV-28 ( Yin jiao ), GV-2 ( Yao shu )

GV-26 treats the low back pain. K-2 eliminates the heat in the kidneys and treats the back pain. BL-40 eliminates the blood stagnation and treats the back pain. BL-60 and GV-28 treat the back pain as distant point. GV-2 is the local point for the back pain. Yao tong xue is the extra acupoint for low back pain. The location is on the dorsum side of the hands, between the third and second metacarpal bones, fourth and fifth metacarpal bones. Bloodletting technique is used on GV-28 and K-2. Strong manipulation is used.

### <239> Acute backpain(2)

There are many different kinds of causes of backpain. Medical consultation is essential. Here in this prescription, we only focus on the pain itself. The GV channel, kidneys and BL channel are the most responsible for the back pain. The local and the distant acupoints are used. It is good to use moving body method when you treat the pain of local area. After needling the distant point, let the patient move the local area of problem. This method will promote the healing process

The main points : GV-20 ( Bai hui ), BL-62 ( Shen mai ), SI-3 ( Hou xi ), Liv-3 ( Tai chong ), GV-26 ( Shui gou )
The accompanying points : Ashi, Yao tong xue ( Ex ), GB-34 ( Yang ling quan )

SI-3 opens the GV channel and needles with BL-62 to treat the back pain. GV-26 treats back pain. Yao tong xue is the extra acupoint for low back pain. The location is on the dorsum side of the hands, between the third and second metacarpal bones, fourth and fifth metacarpal bones. Strong manipulation is used. After needling the hand points, let the patient move the body to release the tension and pain.

### <240> Acute backpain(3)

There are many different kinds of causes of backpain. Medical consultation is essential. Here in this prescription, we only focus on the pain itself. The GV channel, kidneys and BL channel are the most responsible for the back pain. The local and the distant acupoints are used. It is good to use moving body method when you treat the pain of local area. After needling the distant point, let the patient move the local area of problem. This method will promote the healing process

The main points : TB-6 ( Zhi gou ), Liv-3 ( Tai chong ), SP-10 ( Xue hai ), BL-64 ( Jing gu ), GB-34 ( Yang ling quan ), GV-26 ( Shui gou ), K-7 ( Fu liu )
The accompanying points : CV-6 ( Qi hai ), Yao tong xue ( Ex ), GB-12 ( Wan gu ), Lu-5 ( Chi ze ), K-3 ( Tai xi )

Lu-5 relieves the pains on the BL channel of the back. GB-12 relieves the pain on the back. TB-6 opens the TB channel to relieve the stiffness on the thorax. GB-34 relaxes the tendons and muscles.

GV-26 relieves the pain on the back. BL-64 is the distant point for the back pain. CV-6 tonifies the lower burner and Qi. K-7 tonifies the kidneys. Yao tong xue is the extra acupoint for low back pain. The location is on the dorsum side of the hands, between the third and second metacarpal bones, fourth and fifth metacarpal bones. Strong manipulation is used. Let the patient move the back after needling K-7 to release the tension on the back.

### <241> Amyotrophic lateral sclerosis (ALS), Lou Gehrig's disease

Amyotrophic lateral sclerosis (ALS), previously referred to as Lou Gehrig's disease, is a neurological condition that impacts motor neurons. These are the nerve cells located in the brain and spinal cord responsible for governing voluntary muscle movement and breathing. As motor neurons deteriorate and cease to function, they no longer transmit signals to the muscles, resulting in muscle weakness, the onset of muscle twitches, and muscle atrophy. Ultimately, individuals with ALS experience a loss of the brain's capacity to initiate and regulate voluntary activities like chewing, walking, speaking, and various other functions, including breathing. ALS is a progressive ailment and difficult to cure completely. Medical consultation is essential and acupuncture is not a substitute for conventional ALS treatments, but rather a supportive therapy. Early medical consultation is crucial. In TCM view, this issue arises from a deficiency in kidneys essence, which results in the kidneys being unable to adequately nourish the bones, muscles, and nerve. The TCM treatment approach revolves around the concept of replenishing kidney essence.

The main points : K-7 ( Fu liu ), BL-23 ( Shen shu ), GV-4 ( Ming men ), SP-6 ( San yin jiao ), K-6 ( Tai xi ), ST-36 ( Zu san li ), SI-3 ( Hou xi ), CV-4 ( Guan yuan ), CV-6 ( Qi hai ), GB-39 ( Xuan zhong ), BL-18 ( Gan shu ), BL-20 ( Pi shu )

The accompanying points : LI-4 ( He gu ), GV-14 ( Da zhui ), LI-11 ( Qu chi ), LI-10 ( Shou san li ), GB-34 ( Yang ling quan )

Vitamin B injection on 5 points ( practiced in China and some Asian countries only ) : LI-4 ( He gu ), SP-10 ( Xue hai ), Liv-3 ( Tai chong ), ST-36 ( Zu san li ), SP-6 ( San yin jiao ), LI-11 ( Qu chi ), Ba feng ( Ex ), Ba xie ( Ex )

Dang gui ( Angelica sinensis ) liquid injection on 3 points ( practiced in China and some Asian countries only ).

The practice of injecting vitamins or herbal extracts at acupuncture points is generally not permitted in many countries outside of China and some Asian nations. It is advisable to verify the specific acupuncture laws in your own country. Patients are encouraged to actively seek and engage in the treatment.

### <242> Ankle joint pain

The main treatment idea is relaxing and relieving the tension on the local area and treating the inflammation on the tendons and muscles. Medical consultation is essential. The local points and distant points are used. The method of eliminating the dampness is necessary to remove the pain and inflammation.

The main points : ST-36 ( Zu san li ), SP-9 ( Yin ling quan ), GB-40 ( Qiu xu ), Liv-3 ( Tai chong ), ST-43 ( Xian gu ), Ashi, Liv-4 ( Zhong feng ), ST-41 ( Jie xi ), SP-5 ( Shang qiu ), BL-62 ( Shen mai ), K-6 ( Zhao hai ) : it is not necessary to use all these points. You can decide which points to use following the location of pain and diagnosis result.

The accompanying points : GB-41 ( Zu lin qi ), SP-6 ( San yin jiao ), Ht-7 ( Shen men ), SI-4 ( Wan gu ), SI-5 ( Yang gu ), K-8 ( Jiao xin ), BL-65 ( Shu gu )

Ashi points relieves the pain but if the local area is swollen and very painful, the same points but on the opposite side of the body can be needled. SP-6 eliminates the dampness and also removes the blood stagnation. The points of Ht-7, SI-4 or SI-5 are the acupoints on the wrist because the wrist corresponds to the ankle. Strong manipulation is used on acute case. Moxibustion is used on chronic case.

### <243> Ankylosing spondylitis

Ankylosing spondylitis is a form of arthritis characterized by inflammation in the joints and ligaments of the spine. It can also impact peripheral joints such as the knees, ankles, and hips. Individuals with ankylosing spondylitis experience stiffness due to inflammation in the spinal joints and tissues. In severe instances, this condition can lead to the fusion of vertebrae, resulting in a rigid and inflexible spine. Medical consultation is essential. In TCM view, this disease is closely related with deficiency of kidneys Yang, coldness and dampness.

The main points : GV-9 ( Zhi yang ), GV-4 ( Ming men ), BL-23 ( Shen shu ), GV-3 ( Yao yang guan ), GV-14 ( Da zhui ), SP-9 ( Yin ling quan ), Ashi, CV-4 ( Guan yuan ), SI-3 ( Hou xi ), K-7 ( Fu liu ), Jia ji ( Ex )

The accompanying points : GV-16 ( Feng fu ), LI-11 ( Qu chi ), Liv-3 ( Tai chong ), SP-10 ( Xue hai ), Ht-7 ( Shen men ), GV-20 ( Bai hui ), Yin tang ( Ex )

Acupuncture and moxibustion play a certain role in alleviating clinical symptoms and slowing the progression of ankylosing spondylitis, but there is insufficient evidence to suggest that acupuncture and moxibustion can completely cure the disease. TCM herbal medicine is used.

### <244> Bruise, contusion

Bruise has blood stagnation, inflammation and is swollen. Medical consultation is essential. It is necessary to relieve the tension on the local area, remove the blood stagnation, treat the inflammation and dampness to remove the edema. Use the distant points, close points, Ashi points. Strong manipulation is used. Generally the direction of point is towards the pathological place. In case of severe inflammation, needling on Ashi points are prohibited but you can needle on the same points on the opposite side. Bleeding method using cupping on the close points are also effective.

### <245> Chronic backpain

The main treatment idea of chronic backpain is similar to acute backpain but it is necessary to tonify the kidneys and liver because the chronic case is the deficiency of kidneys and liver. You can refer to the section of acute backpain. Medical consultation is essential.

The main points : GV-2 ( Yao shu ), CV-4 ( Guan yuan ) : tonifying method, BL-40 ( Wei zhong ) : bloodletting technique, Shi qi zhui xia ( Ex ), Yao yan ( Ex ), GV-3 ( Yao yang guan )

The accompanying points : Yao tong xue ( Ex ), SI-3 ( Hou xi ), BL-25 ( Da chang shu ), BL-37 ( Yin men ), Ashi, BL-23 ( Shen shu ), BL-22 ( San jiao shu ), BL-26 ( Guan yuan shu )

BL-40 removes the blood stagnation and relieves the tension on the back. BL-37 eliminates the back pain. Shi qi zhui xia is the extra acupoint used for backpain. The location is below the spinous process of the 5th lumbar vertebra. GV-2 is the local point for backpain. The accompanying points are the local points for the backpain. Yao yan is the extra acupoint for the backpain. The location is about 3.5~4 cun lateral to the lower border of the spinous process of the 4th lumbar vertebra. This point is on the depression when the patient is at prone position. Yao tong xue is the extra acupoint for low back pain. The location is on the dorsum side of the hands, between the third and second metacarpal bones, fourth and fifth metacarpal bones. These local points not just relieve the tension on the local area but also have the functions of tonifying kidneys and liver. Moxibustion or needle can be used. Tonifying method is used.

### <246> Cramp in legs, cramp in gastrocnemius

The causes are involuntary nerve discharges, deficiency of blood on legs, stress or too much excessive exercise. The main treatment idea is to relieve the tension on the local area and nourish the blood on the leg. Medical consultation is essential.

The main points : Liv-3 ( Tai chong ), GB-31 ( Feng shi ), K-9 ( Zhu bin ), BL-40 ( Wei zhong ), BL-20 ( Pi shu ), ST-36 ( Zu san li ), BL-57 ( Cheng shan ), BL-56 ( Cheng jin )
The accompanying points : BL-37 ( Yin men ), BL-18 ( Gan shu ), BL-19 ( Dan shu ), BL-60 ( Kun lun ), GB-34 ( Yang ling quan ), SP-6 ( San yin jiao ), BL-23 ( Shen shu ), Ba feng ( Ex )

The local points are used to relieve the tension on the local area. GB-34 relieves the tension on the tendons. ST-36 tonifies Qi and increases the blood circulation on the legs. BL-20 tonifies the spleen and nourishes the blood. BL-23 nourishes the kidneys essence. Ba feng is the extra acupoints on the leg. Ba feng is a group of points at the sides of the toes that relieves the tension on the leg and increases the blood circulation. Strong manipulation is used. Bleeding method on BL-40 can be effective.

### <247> Degenerative arthritis of knee

All degeneration problems happen when the bone is too old and becomes deficient. Medical consultation is essential. In TCM view, the degeneration of bone is due to kidneys deficiency. The main treatment idea is to eliminate the local pain and to nourish the kidneys and liver.

The main points : GB-33 ( Xi yang guan ), PC-3 ( Qu ze ), K-10 ( Yin gu ), BL-40 ( Wei zhong ), Wai xi yan ( Ex ), Nei xi yan ( Ex ), Ashi, ST-36 ( Zu san li ), SP-9 ( Yin ling quan )
The accompanying points : LI-4 ( He gu ), PC-6 ( Nei guan ), Lu-5 ( Chi ze ), SP-10 ( Xue hai ), GB-34 ( Yang ling quan ), SP-6 ( San yin jiao ), ST-34 ( Liang qiu ), Liv-3 ( Tai chong )

LI-4 eliminates the inflammation. Liv-3 is the distant point for the knee pain. Wai xi yan and the Nei xi yan are the extra acupoints for the knee. The locations of Wai xi yan and Nei xi yan are points in the two depressions, medial and lateral to the patellar ligament, locating the point with the knee flexed. The external depression is called Wai xi yan and the internal depression is called Nei xi yan. The local points and distant points are used. SP-10 is the local point but it also nourishes the blood. ST-36 tonifies the Qi and benefits the knees and legs. SP-9 eliminates the dampness and strengthens the spleen. SP-6 nourishes the kidneys Yin to nourish the knee. The acupoints on the elbow like Lu-5 and PC-3 are used because the elbows correspond to the knees. Tonifying manipulation is used. Moxibustion can be effective too.

### <248> Fibromyalgia syndrome ( FMS )

Fibromyalgia is a persistent ailment characterized by enduring discomfort and tenderness distributed throughout the body, coupled with weariness and difficulties in achieving restful sleep. Medical consultation is essential. Although the precise origins of this condition remain incompletely comprehended, individuals afflicted by it exhibit an increased susceptibility to pain, a phenomenon that puzzles scientists. In TCM view, the heart, spleen and kidneys are closely related with this problem. Applying moving cupping therapy along the meridians of the Governing Vessel (GV) and the first line of the Bladder Meridian (BL) is used. The patients can have mental depression.

The main points : GB-34 ( Yang ling quan ), PC-6 ( Nei guan ), BL-20 ( Pi shu ), BL-11 ( Da zhu ), GB-38 ( Yang fu ), BL-18 ( Gan shu ), CV-4 ( Guan yuan ) : the patient concentrate on the feeling of CV-4, CV-3 ( Zhong ji ), moving cupping therapy along the meridians of the GV and BL ( from BL-11 to BL-23 ), Ht-7 ( Shen men ), BL-23 ( Shen shu ), GB-21 ( Jian jing ) : follow the safety guide of acupuncture

The accompanying points : GV-24 ( Shen ting ), CV-12 ( Zhong wan ), GV-20 ( Bai hui ), Ashi, Liv-3 ( Tai chong ), SP-6 ( San yin jiao ), ST-36 ( Zu san li )

The penetrating needle technique is used to increase the therapeutic effects : GB-20 ( Feng chi ) to GV-16 ( Feng fu ) : follow the safety guide of acupuncture, BL-60 ( Kun lun ) to K-6 ( Tai xi ), Yu yao ( Ex ) to GB-14 ( Yang bai ), LI-4 ( He gu ) to Lu-10 ( Yu ji ), PC-6 ( Nei guan ) to TB-5 ( Wai guan ), Tai yang ( Ex ) to TB-23 ( Si zhu kong ), ST-38 ( Tiao kou ) to BL-57 ( Cheng shan ), GB-34 ( Yang ling quan ) to SP-9 ( Yin ling quan )

Moxibustion and electroacupuncture are viable treatment options. Acupuncture manages pain and enhance overall quality of life. TCM herbal medicine is used to enhance the therapeutic effects.

### <249> Frozen shoulder ( Adhesive capsulitis )

Frozen shoulder involves stiffness and pain. Symptoms begin slowly, then they get worse. The main treatment idea is needling the local and distant points. Medical consultation is essential. Most commonly used channels are GB, SI, LI and TB channels that pass the local area.

The main points : TB-3 ( Zhong zhu ), SI-13 ( Qu yuan ), TB-4 ( Yang chi ), SI-12 ( Bing feng ), LI-16 ( Ju gu ), SI-11 ( Tian zong ), GB-21 ( Jian jing ), SI-7 ( Zhi zheng )

The accompanying points : LI-4 ( He gu ), SI-3 ( Hou xi ), GB-34 ( Feng shi ), LI-11 ( Qu chi ), Ashi, TB-15 ( Tian liao ), TB-5 ( Wai guan )

The method of moving shoulder with needles : Needle the acupoints of SP-9 ( Yin ling quan ) and ST-38 ( Tiao kou ) or ST-40 ( Feng long ) and let the patient move the shoulder for a while. This method rapidly relieves the pain and increases the angle of movement.

The local points are used to relieve the local tension. SI-3 is the distant point for the shoulder. LI-11 is the distant point for the shoulder. When you choose the distant point, you can consider which channel passes the local pain area. ST-38 or ST-40 are on the Yang ming channel and it moves blood and Qi intensively and relieves the pains. SP-9 is the He sea point of the SP channel. SP channel and SI channel are connected as special connection. SP-9 can open the SI channel that passes the shoulder. Strong manipulation is used. Bloodletting method on Ashi point can be used.

### <250> Knee joint pain

The local points and the distant points are used together. Medical consultation is essential. Treatment of tendon and muscle is essential. The channels passing through the knee are used commonly.

The main points : ST-36 ( Zu san li ), SP-6 ( San yin jiao ), Ashi, GB-33 ( Xi yang guan ), K-10 ( Yin gu ), Wai xi yan ( Ex ), Nei xi yan ( Ex ), SP-9 ( Yin ling quan ), BL-40 ( Wei zhong )
The accompanying points : ST-34 ( Liang qiu ), Lu-5 ( Chi ze ), PC-3 ( Qu ze ), GB-34 ( Yang ling quan ), SP-10 ( Xue hai ),

ST, SP, SP and BL channels pass through the knee. SP-10 nourishes the blood and tendons. GB-33 is the special point for knee pain. K-10 nourishes the kidneys and also used for knee pain as local point. ST-36 is the essential point for leg pain or knee pain. GB-34 eliminates the dampness from the tendons. BL-40 is the local point of knee and removes the blood stagnation. Wai xi yan and Nei xi yan are the extra acupoints for the knee problems. The locations of Wai xi yan and Nei xi yan are points in the two depressions, medial and lateral to the patellar ligament, locating the point with the knee flexed. The external depression is called Wai xi yan and the internal depression is called Nei xi yan. The acupoints on the inner side of the elbow like Lu-5 and PC-3 are used because the elbows correspond to the knees.

Strong manipulation is used on acute case. Moxibustion is used on chronic case with medium level of needle manipulation.

### <251> Myasthenia gravis

Myasthenia gravis is a persistent autoimmune disorder affecting the neuromuscular system, leading to muscle weakness in the skeletal muscles, which are responsible for bodily movements in the arms and legs, as well as facilitating breathing. Medical consultation is essential. In TCM view, the core symptom of this condition is fatigue and weakness. The main syndrome pattern is the deficiency of spleen and kidneys. The treatment idea should focus on strengthening the spleen and nourishing the kidneys.

The main points : CV-4 ( Guan yuan ), GV-20 ( Bai hui ), CV-6 ( Qi hai ), CV-12 ( Zhong wan ), ST-36 ( Zu san li ), K-7 ( Fu liu ), BL-23 ( Shen shu ), TB-2 ( Ye men ), BL-18 ( Gan shu ), SP-6 ( San yin jiao ), SP-9 ( Yin ling quan ), GV-4 ( Ming men ), SP-10 ( Xue hai )

The accompanying points

For weak eyelids : points around the eyes

For difficulty in swallowing : CV-23 ( Lian quan ), GB-12 ( Wan gu ), GB-20 ( Feng chi ), TB-17 ( Yi feng ), PC-6 ( Nei guan )

For the whole body weakness : GB-30 ( Huan tiao ), BL-40 ( Wei zhong ), LI-4 ( He gu ), Liv-3 ( Tai chong ), TB-5 ( Wai guan ), LI-11 ( Qu chi ), LI-15 ( Jian yu ), GB-34 ( Yang ling quan ),

The constitutional treatment and constitutional diet therapy is used. The TCM herbal medicine is used. The acupoints are mainly about strengthening the spleen, liver and kidneys.

### <252> Raynaud disease

This disease causes mostly the fingers and toes but not limited to these parts. Medical consultation is essential. The patients feel numb and cold in cold temperature or in the stress. In Raynaud's disease, small arteries that send blood to the skin become narrower and it blocks blood flow. The main causes of Raynaud's disease are not known. But other causes seem to be associated with some health problem, such as a rheumatic disease like scleroderma or lupus. Being exposed to coldness or certain chemicals may also cause this disease. In TCM view, this is the stagnation of blood and coldness pattern. The main treatment idea is to eliminate the stagnation of blood and coldness.

The main points : Liv-3 ( Tai chong ), SP-10 ( Xue hai ), BL-18 ( Gan shu ), LI-11 ( Qu chi ), Ba feng ( Ex ), ST-36 ( Zu san li ), GB-38 ( Yang fu ), SP-8 ( Di ji ), Ba xie ( Ex ), PC-4 ( Xi men ), GB-34 ( Yang ling quan ), CV-4 ( Guan yuan )

The accompanying points : TB-4 ( Yang chi ), GV-20 ( Bai hui ), GV-4 ( Ming men ), BL-17 ( Ge shu ), ST-41 ( Jie xi ), K-7 ( Fu liu ), TB-5 ( Wai guan ), BL-23 ( Shen shu )

The local points on fingers and toes are used. Ba xie and Ba feng are the extra acupoints on hands and feet. Ba xie is a group of points at the sides of the fingers. Ba feng is a group of points at the sides of the toes. Ba xie and Ba feng increase the local circulation. BL-18 is the back shu point of liver and removes the blood stagnation. BL-23 is the back shu point of kidneys and tonifies the Kidneys Yang to warm the body and to expel the coldness from the body. SP-8 removes the blood stagnation. BL-17 moves the blood and nourishes the blood. GV-20 tonifies the Qi. GB-34 eliminates the dampness. Needle and moxibustion can be used. The moxibustion can be used to expel the coldness.

### <253> Rheumatoid arthritis ( RA ) - hip joint

This is an autoimmune and inflammatory disease, that is to say, the immune system attacks healthy cells by mistake, and it causes inflammation and the affected local area becomes swollen and painful. Medical consultation is essential. It mainly attacks the joints. In TCM view, this is wind damp heat or wind damp coldness that attacks the local area. The main treatment idea is to regulate the immune system using the points of lung, spleen, kidneys and liver and to eliminate the local pathogens of wind damp heat or wind damp coldness. Usually, the acute case is wind damp heat. In chronic cases, it is necessary to tonify the liver and kidneys at the same time.

The main points : BL-23 ( Shen shu ), ST-31 ( Bi guan ), SP-9 ( Yin ling quan ), BL-32 ( Ci liao ),, CV-4 ( Guan yuan ), BL-52 ( Zhi shi ), ST-36 ( Zu san li ), SP-6 ( San yin jiao ), CV-12 ( Zhong wan ), LI-11 ( Qu chi )

The accompanying points : BL-53 ( Bao huang ), CV-4 ( Guan yuan ), GB-30 ( Huan tiao ), BL-13 ( Fei shu ), BL-20 ( Pi shu ), GB-29 ( Ju liao ), Ashi, GV-4 ( Ming men ), Liv-3 ( Tai chong )

The main points are to regulate the immune system by lung, kidneys and spleen. The accompanying points are to remove the local pathogen on the hip joints. Strong manipulation on the main points, needles, bleeding or moxibustion on the accompanying points for acute case. For the chronic case, the moxibustion or needles with moxibustion ( warm needle technique ) are used.

### <254> Rheumatoid arthritis – Shoulder pain

This is an autoimmune and inflammatory disease, that is to say, the immune system attacks healthy cells by mistake, and it causes inflammation and the affected local area becomes swollen and painful. It mainly attacks the joints. Medical consultation is essential. In TCM view, this is wind damp heat or wind damp coldness that attacks the local area. The main treatment idea is to regulate the immune system using the points of lung, spleen, kidneys and liver and to eliminate the local pathogens of wind damp heat or wind damp coldness. Usually, the acute case is wind damp heat. In chronic cases, it is necessary to tonify the liver and kidneys at the same time.

The main points : BL-23 ( Shen shu ), BL-52 ( Zhi shi ), ST-40 ( Feng long ), Lu-3 ( Tian fu ), TB-14 ( Jian liao ), CV-12 ( Zhong wan

), ST-36 ( Zu san li ), Ht-1 ( Ji quan ), SP-6 ( San yin jiao ), BL-20 ( Pi shu )

The accompanying points : SI-10 ( Nao shu ), LI-4 ( He gu ), CV-4 ( Guan yuan ), Ashi, TB-13 ( Nao hui ), LI-15 ( Jian yu ), LI-16 ( Ju gu ), BL-13 ( Fei shu ), SI-3 ( Hou xi )

The main points are to regulate the immune system by lung, kidneys and spleen. The accompanying points are to remove the local pathogen on the local area. Strong manipulation on the main points, needles, bleeding or moxibustion on the accompanying points for acute case. For the chronic case, the moxibustion or needles with moxibustion ( Warm needle technique ) are used.

### <255> Rheumatoid arthritis – elbows

This is an autoimmune and inflammatory disease, that is to say, the immune system attacks healthy cells by mistake, and it causes inflammation and the affected local area becomes swollen and painful. It mainly attacks the joints. Medical consultation is essential. In TCM view, this is wind damp heat or wind damp coldness that attacks the local area. The main treatment idea is to regulate the immune system using the points of lung, spleen, kidneys and liver and to eliminate the local pathogens of wind damp heat or wind damp coldness. Usually, the acute case is wind damp heat. In chronic cases, it is necessary to tonify the liver and kidneys at the same time.

The main points : ST-36 ( Zu san li ), Lu-5 ( Chi ze ), Liv-3 ( Tai chong ), SP-10 ( Xue hai ), SI-8 ( Xiao hai ), BL-20 ( Pi shu ), SP-6 ( San yin jiao ), BL-13 ( Fei shu ), CV-4 ( Guan yuan ), TB-10 ( Tian jing ), LI-12 ( Zhou liao )

The accompanying points : BL-52 ( Zhi shi ), Ashi, ST-40 ( Feng long ), CV-12 ( Zhong wan ), BL-23 ( Shen shu ), LI-4 ( He gu ), PC-3 ( Qu ze ), Ht-3 ( Shao hai ), LI-11 ( Qu chi )

The main points are to regulate the immune system by lung, kidneys and spleen. The accompanying points are to remove the local pathogen on the local area. Strong manipulation on the main points, needles, bleeding or moxibustion on the accompanying points for acute case. For the chronic case, the moxibustion or needles with moxibustion ( Warm needle technique ) are used.

### <256> Rheumatoid arthritis – finger

This is an autoimmune and inflammatory disease, that is to say, the immune system attacks healthy cells by mistake, and it causes inflammation and the affected local area becomes swollen and painful. Medical consultation is essential. It mainly attacks the joints. In TCM view, this is wind damp heat or wind damp coldness that attacks the local area. The main treatment idea is to regulate the immune system using the points of lung, spleen, kidneys and liver and to eliminate the local pathogens of wind damp heat or wind damp coldness. Usually, the acute case is wind damp heat. In chronic cases, it is necessary to tonify the liver and kidneys at the same time.

The main points : BL-23 ( Shen shu ), BL-13 ( Fei shu ), Liv-3 ( Tai chong ), BL-20 ( Pi shu ), BL-52 ( Zhi shi ), ST-36 ( Zu san li ), Lu-9 ( Tai yuan ), SP-10 ( Xue hai ), Ashi, CV-4 ( Guan yuan ), Ba xie ( Ex )

The accompanying points : TB-4 ( Yang chi ), GB-34 ( Yang ling quan ), LI-4 ( He gu ), SP-6 ( San yin jiao ), CV-12 ( Zhong wan ), LI-5 ( Yang xi ), GB-31 ( Feng shi ), PC-7 ( Da ling ), SI-4 ( Wan gu ), Ht-7 ( Shen men )

The main points are to regulate the immune system by lung, kidneys and spleen. The accompanying points are to remove the local pathogen on the local area. Strong manipulation on the main points, needles, bleeding or moxibustion on the accompanying points for acute case. For the chronic case, the moxibustion or needles with moxibustion ( Warm needle technique ) are used.

<257> **Rheumatoid arthritis – knee**

This is an autoimmune and inflammatory disease, that is to say, the immune system attacks healthy cells by mistake, and it causes inflammation and the affected local area becomes swollen and painful. It mainly attacks the joints. Medical consultation is essential. In TCM view, this is wind damp heat or wind damp coldness that attacks the local area. The main treatment idea is to regulate the immune system using the points of lung, spleen, kidneys and liver and to eliminate the local pathogens of wind damp heat or wind damp coldness. Usually, the acute case is wind damp heat. In chronic cases, it is necessary to tonify the liver and kidneys at the same time.

The main points : SP-9 ( Yin ling quan ), BL-23 ( Shen shu ), Nei xi yan ( Ex ), Wai xi yan ( Ex ), CV-4 ( Guan yuan ), BL-13 ( Fei shu ), BL-20 ( Pi shu ), ST-36 ( Zu san li ), SP-6 ( San yin jiao ), Ashi, P-5 ( Chi ze ), PC-3 ( Qu ze )

The accompanying points : ST-34 ( Liang qiu ), ST-40 ( Feng long ), BL-52 ( Zhi shi ), CV-12 ( Zhong wan ), He ding ( Ex ), GB-34 ( Yang ling quan ), BL-40 ( Wei zhong ) : bloodletting technique

The main points are to regulate the immune system by lung, kidneys and spleen. The accompanying points are to remove the local pathogen on the local area. Strong manipulation on the main points, needles, bleeding or moxibustion on the accompanying points for acute case. Wai xi yan and Nei xi yan are the extra acupoints for the knee. Wai xi yan and Nei xi yan are the extra acupoints for the knee problems. The locations of Wai xi yan and Nei xi yan are points in the two depressions, medial and lateral to the patellar ligament, locating the point with the knee flexed. The external depression is called Wai xi yan and the internal depression is called Nei xi yan. He ding is the extra acupoint for the knee problems. The location is above the knee, in the depression of the midpoint of the superior patellar border of knee. For the chronic case, the moxibustion or needles with moxibustion ( warm needle technique ) are used.

### <258> Rheumatoid inflammation of ankle joint

This is an autoimmune and inflammatory disease, that is to say, the immune system attacks healthy cells by mistake, and it causes inflammation and the affected local area becomes swollen and painful. It mainly attacks the joints. Medical consultation is essential. In TCM view, this is wind damp heat or wind damp coldness that attacks the local area. The main treatment idea is to regulate the immune system using the points of lung, spleen, kidneys and liver and to eliminate the local pathogens of wind damp heat or wind damp coldness. Usually, the acute case is wind damp heat. In chronic cases, it is necessary to tonify the liver and kidneys at the same time.

The main points : BL-23 ( Shen shu ), Lu-9 ( Tai yuan ), ST-41 ( Jie xi ), Liv-4 ( Zhong feng ), BL-20 ( Pi shu ), ST-36 ( Zu san li ), SP-6 ( San yin jiao ), CV-4 ( Guan yuan ), K-3 ( Tai xi ), BL-62 ( Shen mai ), BL-13 ( Fei shu )

The accompanying points : GB-34 ( Yang ling quan ), GB-40 ( Qiu xu ), SI-5 ( Yang gu ), BL-52 ( Zhi shi ), CV-12 ( Zhong wan ), K-6 ( Zhao hai ), Ashi

The main points are to regulate the immune system by lung, kidneys and spleen. The accompanying points are to remove the local pathogen on the local area. Strong manipulation on the main points, needles, bleeding or moxibustion on the accompanying points for acute case. For the chronic case, the moxibustion or needles with moxibustion ( Warm needle technique ) are used.

### <259> Rheumatoid pain of muscles

This is an autoimmune and inflammatory disease, that is to say, the immune system attacks healthy cells by mistake, and it causes inflammation and the affected local area becomes swollen and painful. It mainly attacks the joints. Medical consultation is essential. In TCM view, this is wind damp heat or wind damp coldness that attacks the local area. The main treatment idea is to regulate the immune system using the points of lung, spleen, kidneys and liver and to eliminate the local pathogens of wind damp heat or wind damp coldness. Usually, the acute case is wind damp heat. In chronic cases, it is necessary to tonify the liver and kidneys at the same time.

The main points : BL-15 ( Xin shu ), SP-10 ( Xue hai ), LI-4 ( He gu ), BL-20 ( Pi shu ), SP-6 ( San yin jiao ), GV-20 ( Bai hui ), ST-36 ( Zu san li ), CV-4 ( Guan yuan ), BL-23 ( Shen shu ), Liv-3 ( Tai chong )

The accompanying points : GB-34 ( Yang ling quan ), BL-18 ( Gan shu ), Ashi

The main points are to regulate the immune system by lung, kidneys and spleen. The accompanying points are to remove the local pathogen on the local area. Strong manipulation is used on the main points. Bleeding method by cupping or magnets can be used on the Ashi points.

### <260> Rheumatoid temporomandibular disorder

This is an autoimmune and inflammatory disease, that is to say, the immune system attacks healthy cells by mistake, and it causes inflammation and the affected local area becomes swollen and painful. It mainly attacks the joints. Medical consultation is essential. In TCM view, this is wind damp heat or wind damp coldness that attacks the local area. The main treatment idea is to regulate the immune system using the points of lung, spleen, kidneys and liver and to eliminate the local pathogens of wind damp heat or wind damp coldness. Usually, the acute case is wind damp heat. In chronic cases, it is necessary to tonify the liver and kidneys at the same time.

The main points : BL-23 ( Shen shu ), ST-7 ( Xia guan ), SI-19 ( Ting gong ), Qian zheng ( Ex ), Liv-3 ( Tai chong ), SP-6 ( San yin jiao ), BL-20 ( Pi shu ), BL-15 ( Xin shu ), GV-20 ( Bai hui )

The accompanying points : GB-34 ( Yang ling quan ), SI-17 ( Tian rong ), LI-4 ( He gu ), CV-4 ( Guan yuan ), GB-20 ( Feng chi ), GB-2 ( Ting hui ), Ashi

The main points are to regulate the immune system by lung, kidneys and spleen. The accompanying points are to remove the local pathogen on the local area. Strong manipulation on the main points, needles, bleeding or moxibustion on the accompanying points for acute case. For the chronic case, the moxibustion or needles with moxibustion ( Warm needle technique ) are used.

### <261> Shoulder and arm pain

There are many causes of shoulder and arm pain. But here we focus on the treatment of pain itself. Medical consultation is essential. If any causes are known, it is necessary to eliminate those causes. The main treatment idea is to regulate the Qi and blood of the local affected area using the local and distant points.

The main points : LI-4 ( He gu ), PC-6 ( Nei guan ), SI-11 ( Tian zong ), TB-15 ( Tian liao ), LI-11 ( Qu chi ), TB-13 ( Nao hui ), SI-5 ( Zhi zheng ), LI-10 ( Shou san li )

The accompanying points : LI-14 ( Bi nao ), TA-14 ( Jian liao ), LI-15 ( Jian yu ), TB-5 ( Wai guan ), SI-10 ( Nao shu ), SI-15 ( Jian Zhong shu ), LI-16 ( Ju gu )

The other method : ST-38 ( Tiao kou ) or ST-40 ( Feng long ), or SP-9 ( Yin ling quan ) ( Aftter deep needling, let the patient move their shoulder and it relieves the pain of shoulder )

The local and distant points are used to regulate the Qi and blood on the local area. TB, LI and SI channels are used commonly because they pass through the shoulder and arms. If the local area is too painful and it is difficult to needle there, needling on the opposite side is also possible. Strong manipulation is used. Bleeding method can be used near the Ashi points.

### <262> Shoulder joint pain

There are many causes of shoulder joint pain. But here we focus on the treatment of pain itself. Medical consultation is essential. If any causes are known, it is necessary to eliminate those causes. The main treatment idea is to regulate the Qi and blood of the local affected area using the local and distant points.

The main points : SI-7 ( Zhi zheng ), Ht-8 ( Shao fu ) : use reducing method, SI-12 ( Bing feng ), Ashi, LI-16 ( Ju gu ), LI-15 ( Jian yu ), TB-14 ( Jian liao ), SI-10 ( Nao shu ), ST-38 ( Tiao kou ) : deep needling more than 2.5 cun

The accompanying points : GB-21 ( Jiang zheng ), TB-3 ( Zhong zhu ), TB-6 ( Zhi gou ), Ht-1 ( Ji quan ) : do not use thick needle and do not needle fast, there is a danger of hurting the blood vessels, LI-11 ( Qu chi ), SI-11 ( Tian zong ), LI-14 ( Bi nao )

The other method : ST-38 ( Tiao kou ) or ST-40 ( Feng long ), or SP-9 ( Yin ling quan ) ( After deep needling, let the patient move their shoulder and it relieves the pain )

The local and distant points are used to regulate the Qi and blood on the local area. TB, LI and SI channels are used commonly because they pass through the shoulder and arms. If the local area is too painful and it is difficult to needle there, needling on the opposite side is also possible. Strong manipulation on the main points, needles, bleeding or moxibustion on the accompanying points for acute case. For the chronic case, the moxibustion or needles with moxibustion ( warm needle technique ) are used.

### <263> Sprain

All sprains have local blood stagnation. If the local area is swollen and painful, you shouldn't needle the local points. Medical consultation is essential. Instead, the opposite side or the distant points can be used. After the pain get better, you can needle the local area. Point selection methods of distance points, close points and Ashi points can be used. Usually if there is a severe pain and locally swollen, it is better not use the local pain points. Instead, the distance points and close points can be used. The points on the opposite side of the painful side can be used. The corresponding points or the same family channels can be used. The detail explanations are shown below on each section. In treatment of pain, usually let the patient move a little the local painful area after needling the corresponding channels or distant points. It usually relieves the pain faster. But in case of sprain, usually the patients have difficulty in moving the local pain area because the sprain is too painful or because of edema. In that case, it is not necessary to let the patient move the local area.

### <264> Sprain of elbow or knee joints (1)

Medical consultation is essential.

The main points : LI-4 ( He gu ), ST-36 ( Zu san li ), ST-35 ( Du bi ), LI-11 ( Qu chi )

The accompanying points : You can use other acupoints to eliminate the blood stagnation and Ashi points. Liv-3 ( Tai chong ), SP-10 ( Xue hai ), ST-40 ( Feng long ) : bloodletting technique

If there is sprain of elbow, you can choose the point on the knee ( ST-35 ) and if there is sprain of knee, you can choose the point on the elbow ( LI-11 ). It is because the two areas of elbow and knee are corresponding each other. And ST channel and LI channel are the same family channel as Yang ming channel. The direction of needle is to the pain points. Strong manipulation is used. The patient moves the local area after the needles are removed to release the local tension. Here the six prescriptions for sprain of elbow or knee joints ( 1 – 6 ) are shown. Considering the location of pain and the affected channels, you can choose the proper prescription.

### <265> Sprain of elbow or knee joints (2)

Medical consultation is essential.

The main points : LI-4 ( He gu ), ST-36 ( Zu san li ), SP-9 ( Yin ling quan ), Lu-5 ( Chi ze )

The accompanying points : You can use other acupoints to eliminate the blood stagnation and Ashi points. Liv-3 ( Tai chong ), SP-10 ( Xue hai ), ST-40 ( Feng long ) : bloodletting technique

If there is sprain of elbow, you can choose the point on the knee ( SP-9 ) and if there is sprain of knee, you can choose the point on the elbow ( Lu-5 ). It is because the two areas of elbow and knee are corresponding each other. And Lu channel and SP channel are the same family channel as Tai yin channel. The direction of needle is to the pain points. Strong manipulation is used. The patient moves the local area after the needles are removed to release the local tension. Here the six prescriptions for sprain of elbow or knee joints ( 1 – 6 ) are shown. Considering the location of pain and the affected channels, you can choose the proper prescription.

### <266> Sprain of elbow or knee joints (3)

Medical consultation is essential.

The main points : LI-4 ( He gu ), ST-36 ( Zu san li ), GB-34 ( Yang ling quan ), TB-10 ( Tian jing )

The accompanying points : You can use other acupoints to eliminate the blood stagnation and Ashi points. Liv-3 ( Tai chong ), SP-10 ( Xue hai ), ST-40 ( Feng long ) : bloodletting technique

If there is sprain of elbow, you can choose the point on the knee ( GB-34 ) and if there is sprain of knee, you can choose the point on the elbow ( TB-10 ). It is because the two areas of elbow and knee are corresponding each other. And GB channel and TB channel are the same family channel as Shao yang channel. The direction of needle is to the pain points. Strong manipulation is used. The patient moves the local area after the needles are removed to release the local tension. Here the six prescriptions for sprain of elbow or knee joints ( 1 –

6 ) are shown. Considering the location of pain and the affected channels, you can choose the proper prescription.

### <267> Sprain of elbow or knee joints (4)

Medical consultation is essential.

The main points : LI-4 ( He gu ), ST-36 ( Zu san li ), Liv-8 ( Qu quan ), PC-3 ( Qu ze )

The accompanying points : You can use other acupoints to eliminate the blood stagnation and Ashi points. Liv-3 ( Tai chong ), SP-10 ( Xue hai ), ST-40 ( Feng long ) : bloodletting technique

If there is sprain of elbow, you can choose the point on the knee ( Liv-8 ) and if there is sprain of knee, you can choose the point on the elbow ( PC-3 ). It is because the two areas of elbow and knee are corresponding each other. And Liv channel and PC channel are the same family channel as Jue yin channel. The direction of needle is to the pain points. Strong manipulation is used. The patient moves the local area after the needles are removed to release the local tension. Here the six prescriptions for sprain of elbow or knee joints ( 1 – 6 ) are shown. Considering the location of pain and the affected channels, you can choose the proper prescription.

### <268> Sprain of elbow or knee joints (5)

Medical consultation is essential.

The main points : LI-4 ( He gu ), ST-36 ( Zu san li ), BL-40 ( Wei zhong ), SI-8 ( Xiao hai )

The accompanying points : You can use other acupoints to eliminate the blood stagnation and Ashi points. Liv-3 ( Tai chong ), SP-10 ( Xue hai ), ST-40 ( Feng long ) : bloodletting technique

If there is sprain of elbow, you can choose the point on the knee ( BL-40 ) and if there is sprain of knee, you can choose the point on the elbow ( SI-8 ). It is because the two areas of elbow and knee are corresponding each other. And BL channel and SI channel are the same family channel as Tai yang channel. The direction of needle is to the pain points. Strong manipulation is used. The patient moves the local area after the needles are removed to release the local tension. Here the six prescriptions for sprain of elbow or knee joints ( 1 – 6 ) are shown. Considering the location of pain and the affected channels, you can choose the proper prescription.

### <269> Sprain of elbow or knee joints (6)

Medical consultation is essential.

The main points : LI-4 ( He gu ), ST-36 ( Zu san li ), K-10 ( Yin gu ), Ht-3 ( Shao hai )

The accompanying points : You can use other acupoints to eliminate the blood stagnation and Ashi points. Liv-3 ( Tai chong ), SP-10 ( Xue hai ), ST-40 ( Feng long ) : bloodletting technique

If there is sprain of elbow, you can choose the point on the knee ( K-10 ) and if there is sprain of knee, you can choose the point on the elbow ( Ht-3 ). It is because the two areas of elbow and knee are corresponding each other. And K channel and Ht channel are the same family channel as Shao yin channel. The direction of needle is to the pain points. Strong manipulation is used. The patient moves the local area after the needles are removed to release the local tension. Here the six prescriptions for sprain of elbow or knee joints ( 1 – 6 ) are shown. Considering the location of pain and the affected channels, you can choose the proper prescription.

### <270> Sprain of wrist or ankle (1)

Medical consultation is essential.

The main points : LI-4 ( He gu ), SP-6 ( San yin jiao ), GB-40 ( Qiu xu ), TB-4 ( Yang chi )

The accompanying points : You can use other acupoints to eliminate the blood stagnation and Ashi points. Liv-3 ( Tai chong ), SP-10 ( Xue hai ), ST-40 ( Feng long ) : bloodletting technique

If there is sprain of wrist, you can choose the point on the ankle ( GB-40 ) and if there is sprain of ankle, you can choose the point on the wrist ( TB-4 ). It is because the two areas of wrist and ankle are corresponding each other. And GB channel and TB channel are the same family channel as Shao yang channel. The direction of needle is to the pain points. Strong manipulation is used. The patient moves the local area after the needles are removed to release the local tension. Here the six prescriptions for sprain of wrist or ankle joints ( 1 – 6 ) are shown. Considering the location of pain and the affected channels, you can choose the proper prescription.

### <271> Sprain of wrist or ankle (2)

Medical consultation is essential.

The main points : LI-4 ( He gu ), SP-6 ( San yin jiao ), Lu-9 ( Tai yuan ), SP-5 ( Shang qiu )

The accompanying points : You can use other acupoints to eliminate the blood stagnation and Ashi points. Liv-3 ( Tai chong ), SP-10 ( Xue hai ), ST-40 ( Feng long ) : bloodletting technique

If there is sprain of wrist, you can choose the point on the ankle ( SP-5 ) and if there is sprain of ankle, you can choose the point on the wrist ( Lu-9 ). It is because the two areas of wrist and ankle are corresponding each other. And SP channel and Lu channel are the same family channel as Tai yin channel. The direction of needle is to the pain points. Strong manipulation is used. The patient moves the local area after the needles are removed to release the local tension. Here the six prescriptions for sprain of wrist or ankle joints ( 1 – 6 ) are shown. Considering the location of pain and the affected channels, you can choose the proper prescription.

### <272> Sprain of wrist or ankle (3)

Medical consultation is essential.

The main points : LI-4 ( He gu ), SP-6 ( San yin jiao ), ST-41 ( Jie xi ), LI-5 ( Yang xi )

The accompanying points : You can use other acupoints to eliminate the blood stagnation and Ashi points. Liv-3 ( Tai chong ), SP-10 ( Xue hai ), ST-40 ( Feng long ) : bloodletting technique

If there is sprain of wrist, you can choose the point on the ankle ( ST-41 ) and if there is sprain of ankle, you can choose the point on the wrist ( LI-5 ). It is because the two areas of wrist and ankle are corresponding each other. And ST channel and LI channel are the same family channel as Yang ming channel. The direction of needle is to the pain points. Strong manipulation is used. The patient moves the local area after the needles are removed to release the local tension. Here the six prescriptions for sprain of wrist or ankle joints ( 1 - 6 ) are shown. Considering the location of pain and the affected channels, you can choose the proper prescription.

### <273> Sprain of wrist or ankle (4)

Medical consultation is essential.

The main points : LI-4 ( He gu ), SP-6 ( San yin jiao ), Liv-4 ( Zhong feng ), PC-7 ( Da ling )

The accompanying points : You can use other acupoints to eliminate the blood stagnation and Ashi points. Liv-3 ( Tai chong ), SP-10 ( Xue hai ), ST-40 ( Feng long ) : bloodletting technique

If there is sprain of wrist, you can choose the point on the ankle ( Liv-4 ) and if there is sprain of ankle, you can choose the point on the wrist ( PC-7 ). It is because the two areas of wrist and ankle are corresponding each other. And Liv channel and PC channel are the same family channel as Jue yin channel. The direction of needle is to the pain points. Strong manipulation is used. The patient moves the local area after the needles are removed to release the local tension. Here the six prescriptions for sprain of wrist or ankle joints ( 1 - 6 ) are shown. Considering the location of pain and the affected channels, you can choose the proper prescription.

### <274> Sprain of wrist or ankle (5)

Medical consultation is essential.

The main points : LI-4 ( He gu ), SP-6 ( San yin jiao ), BL-60 ( Kun lun ), SI-5 ( Yang gu )

The accompanying points : You can use other acupoints to eliminate the blood stagnation and Ashi points. Liv-3 ( Tai chong ), SP-10 ( Xue hai ), ST-40 ( Feng long ) : bloodletting technique

If there is sprain of wrist, you can choose the point on the ankle ( BL-60 ) and if there is sprain of ankle, you can choose the point on the wrist ( SI-5 ). It is because the two areas of wrist and ankle are corresponding each other. And BL channel and SI channel are the same family channel as Tai yang channel. The direction of needle is to the pain points. Strong manipulation is used. The patient moves the local area after the needles are removed to release the local tension. Here the six prescriptions for sprain of wrist or ankle joints ( 1 – 6 ) are shown. Considering the location of pain and the affected channels, you can choose the proper prescription.

### <275> Sprain of wrist or ankle (6)

Medical consultation is essential.

The main points : LI-4 ( He gu ), SP-6 ( San yin jiao ), K-3 ( Tai xi ), Ht-7 ( Shen men )

The accompanying points : You can use other acupoints to eliminate the blood stagnation and Ashi points. Liv-3 ( Tai chong ), SP-10 ( Xue hai ), ST-40 ( Feng long ) : bloodletting technique

If there is sprain of wrist, you can choose the point on the ankle ( K-3 ) and if there is sprain of ankle, you can choose the point on the wrist ( Ht-7 ). It is because the two areas of wrist and ankle are corresponding each other. And K channel and Ht channel are the same family channel as Shao yin channel. The direction of needle is to the pain points. Strong manipulation is used. The patient moves the local area after the needles are removed to release the local tension. Here the six prescriptions for sprain of wrist or ankle joints ( 1 – 6 ) are shown. Considering the location of pain and the affected channels, you can choose the proper prescription.

### <276> Stiff neck

Stiff neck usually result from injury, sleeping in wrong position or overuse. Medical consultation is essential. Massage, warm or cold packs can relieve it but there are severe cases such as meningitis. The prescription here is to relieve the tension on the local area and relive the pain itself.

The main points : Liv-3 ( Tai chong ), TB-5 ( Wai guan ), Wai lao gong ( Ex ), SI-3 ( Hou xi ), GB-41 ( Zu lin qi ), GB-34 ( Yang ling quan )

The accompanying points : BL-60 ( Kun lun ), BL-10 ( Tian zhu ), TB-16 ( Tian you ), SI-6 ( Yang lao ), GB-20 ( Feng chi ), GV-26 ( Shui gou )

The other method : After needling Wai lao gong ( Ex ), Liv-3 ( Tai chong ) and SI-6 ( Yang lao ), let the patient move the neck to relieve the tension.

Wai lao gong is the extra acupoint for the neck pain. The location is on the dorsal side of the point, PC-8 ( Lao gong ). SI-3 opens the channel of GV that passes the neck. TB-5 relieves the neck pain through opening the TB channel that passes the neck. GB-41 is the distant point for the neck pain. BL-10 is the local point for the neck pain and it relieves the pain. GV-26 opens the GV channel to treat the vertebrae. GB-20 relieves the local pain of the neck. TB-16 is the local point of neck. SI-6 is the Xi cleft point of SI channel and it relieves the neck pain. Let the patient move the neck after the distance points are needled. The strong manipulation is used on Wai lao gong. After the movement of neck is over, needle the close points.

### <277> Suppurative arthritis of knee ( Septic arthritis of knee )

This is a painful infection in a knee joint. The causes are germs that travel through the bloodstream. Medical consultation is essential. It can occur when the patient had an animal bite or trauma, that delivers germs into the joint. The main treatment idea is to eliminate the local inflammation and pathogens. Usually the local and distant points are used to regulate the local area.

The main points : LI-11 ( Qu chi ), Liv-7 ( Xi guan ), PC-3 ( Qu ze ), GB-34 ( Yang ling quan ), Nei xi yan ( Ex ), Wai xi yan ( Ex ), He ding ( Ex ), Liv-8 ( Qu quan ), Lu-5 ( Chi ze )

The accompanying points : LI-4 ( He gu ), K-10 ( Yin gu ), BL-40 ( Wei zhong ) : bloodletting technique, ST-44 ( Nei ting ), ST-34 ( Liang qiu ), GB-33 ( Xi yang guan ), ST-36 ( Zu san li ), SP-10 ( Xue hai ), SP-6 ( San yin jiao ), BL-11 ( Da zhu ), ST-38 ( Tiao kou ) : bloodletting technique

BL-11 benefits the bones and joints and also eliminates the pathogens. Wai xi yan and Nei xi yan are the extra acupoints for the knee problems. The locations of Wai xi yan and Nei xi yan are points in the two depressions, medial and lateral to the patellar ligament, locating the point with the knee flexed. The external depression is called Wai xi yan and the internal depression is called Nei xi yan. He ding is the extra acupoint for the knee problems. The location is above the knee, in the depression of the midpoint of the superior patellar border of knee. ST-36 eliminates the dampness and relieves the knee pain. GB-34 eliminates the dampness on the tendon. K-10 relieves the knee pain and also strengthens the kidneys and bones. Liv-8 is the local point and also strengthens the liver and tendon. SP-10 is the local point and moves the blood. ST-34 is the local point and relieves the knee pain. Liv-7 is the extra acupoint for knee problems. SP-6 eliminates the dampness and nourishes the kidneys and liver. GB-33 is the local point. The strong manipulation is used. Remove the needles immediately after the manipulation. Moxibustion on the Wai xi yan and Nei xi yan can be used to eliminate the local inflammation.

### <278> Suppurative inflammation of ankle joint ( Septic arthritis of ankle joint )

This is a painful infection in an ankle joint. The causes are germs that travel through the bloodstream. Medical consultation is essential. It can occur when the patient had an animal bite or trauma, that delivers germs into the joint. The main treatment idea is to eliminate the local inflammation and pathogens. Usually the local and distant points are used to regulate the local area.

The main points : LI-11 ( Qu chi ), BL-62 ( Shen mai ), GB-40 ( Qiu xu ), SP-6 ( San yin jiao ), BL-59 ( Fu yang ), BL-60 ( Kun lun ), Liv-4 ( Zhong feng ), Liv-6 ( Zhong du ), SP-5 ( Shang qiu ), ST-41 ( Jie xi )

The accompanying points : LI-4 ( He gu ), K-6 ( Zhao hai ), ST-44 ( Nei ting ), K-3 ( Tai xi ), ST-38 ( Tiao kou ), K-7 ( Fu liu ), Liv-3 ( Tai chong ), ST-43 ( Xian gu ), GB-39 ( Xuan zhong )

The local points and distant points are used. The SP, Liv, GB, ST and K channels that pass the ankle are used mostly. The strong manipulation is used. Remove the needles immediately after the manipulation. Moxibustion can be used to eliminate the local inflammation.

### <279> Tennis elbow ( lateral epicondylitis )

This is tearing or swelling of the tendons that are used when you bend the wrist backward from the palm. Medical consultation is essential. The main causes are repetitive motions of the forearm attached to the external part of elbow. The patient experiences the soreness and excessive strain on the local area. LI and ST channels are used mostly because they are the channels that pass through the local painful area.

The main points : ST-36 ( Zu san li ), Ashi, Lu-5 ( Chi ze ) : bloodletting technique, LI-11 ( Qu chi ), LI-10 ( Shou san li ), TB-10( Tian jing ), LI-14 ( Bi nao )

The accompanying points : BL-40 ( Wei zhong ) : bloodletting technique, TB-5 ( Wai guan ), LI-4 ( He gu ), ST-38 ( Tiao kou ), LI-12 ( Zhou liao )

The other method : ST-36 ( Zu san li ), ST-37 ( Shang ju xu ), needle these points around the Yang ming channel on the leg and let the patient move the local area. This area on the leg corresponds to the pain area of forearm.

LI-11 eliminates the local inflammation. LI-12 is the local point. Lu-5 reduces the tension and heat of the local area. Ashi point regulates the local area. LI-4 eliminates the inflammation and heat and it is also the distant point. Other points are all local and distant points. The strong manipulation is used of the main points and Ashi

### <280> Tenosynovitis of index finger

This is an inflammation of the synovial membrane. The patients experience the pain and have a difficulty in moving. Medical consultation is essential. There are infection and non-infection types. The main treatment idea is to regulate the Qi and blood on the local area and to promote the recovery. It is good to treat it in an occidental medicine and TCM way at the same time.

The main points : The two points of Ba xie ( Ex ) near the index finger, LI-11 ( Qu chi ), TB-4 ( Yang chi ), LI-4 ( He gu ), TB-5 ( Wai guan )

The accompanying points : ST-44 ( Nei ting ), Liv-2 ( Xing jian ), Ashi, LI-10 ( Shou san li ), LI-5 ( Yang xi )

LI-11, LI-10 and TB-5 are the distant points to regulate the Qi and blood. LI-5, TB-4 and LI-4 are the local points. ST-44 and Liv-2 are used because the fingers correspond to the toes. The strong manipulation is used for the main points. Ba xie is a group of points at the sides of the fingers on the dorsal side of hand. The intradermal needle or seven star needle ( cutaneous needle ) can be used for the Ashi points.

### <281> Thumb tenosynovitis

This is an inflammation of the synovial membrane. The patients experience the pain and have a difficulty in moving. Medical consultation is essential. There are infection and non-infection types. The main treatment idea is to regulate the Qi and blood on the local area and to promote the recovery. It is good to treat it in an occidental medicine and TCM way at the same time.

The main points : The two points of Ba xie ( Ex ) near the thumb, Lu-5 ( Chi ze ), SP-9 ( Yin ling quan ), Lu-10 ( Yu ji ), LI-5 ( Yang xi )
The accompanying points : SP-6 ( San yin jiao ), LI-10 ( Shou san li ), SP-2 ( Da du ), Lu-9 ( Tai yuan ), Lu-6 ( Kong zui ), Ashi

Lu-5, Lu-6, LI-10 are the distant point. Lu-9, Lu-10 and LI-5 are the local points. The strong manipulation is used for the main points. The SP channel is the same family with Lu channel as Tai yin channel family and the thumb is where the Lu channel is passing. SP-9 eliminates the dampness on the articulations. The intradermal needle or seven star needle ( cutaneous needle ) can be used for the accompanying points.

### <282> Upper arm pain

There are many causes of upper arm pain. If any cause is known, it is necessary to treat that cause. Medical consultation is essential. In this prescription, we focus on the treatment of pain regulating the Qi and blood of the local area. The local and distant points are used.

The main points : SI-7 ( Zhi zheng ), ST-38 ( Tiao kou ), TB-9 ( Si du ), SI-3 ( Hou xi ), Jia ji ( Ex ) of C4~C7 and T1, Lu-5 ( Chi ze ), LI-4 ( He gu ), GB-34 ( Yang ling quan )

The accompanying points : Liv-3 ( Tai chong ), SI-11 ( Tian zong ), Ht-3 ( Shao hai ), LI-11 ( Qu chi ), SI-10 ( Nao shu ), TB-13 ( Nao hui ), SP-9 ( Yin ling quan ), TB-14 ( Bi nao ), TB-5 ( Wai guan )

Jia ji is the extra acupoints on both sides of vertebrae. Depending on the local pain area, the points of Jia ji can be selected. In this prescription, the Jia ji points of C4~C7 and T1 that correspond to the upper arms are used. The local and distant points are used to regulate the Qi and blood of the local area. The Jia ji points are needled at the painful side with deep needling until the patients have the feeling of De Qi on their hands. The strong manipulation is used.

### <283> Wrist ganglion or ankle ganglion ( Ganglion cysts )

Ganglion cysts most often appear on the tendons, wrist joints or hands. But it also occurs in feet or ankle. Medical consultation is essential. This is benign cysts and usually are filled with a jellylike fluid. In TCM way, just needling on the Ashi points makes the holes on the cysts and the fluid of cysts are absorbed inside and the cysts can disappear.

The main points : Ashi ( on the cysts )

The accompanying points : ST-40 ( Feng long ), Liv-3 ( Tai chong ), SP-10 ( Xue hai )

The other method: After you make a hole on the cysts with a thick needle, squeeze out the fluids of the cysts by pressing it. It removes the cysts immediately.

If the ganglion is full of fluids, it will be absorbed through the needle hole of the Ashi. The needle with moxibustion can be used on the Ashi points. The method of squeezing out the fluids can be used after you make a hole on the cysts with a thick needle. Usually the five needles from the five different directions are used on the Ashi ( 4 different directions like front, back, left and right added with the top ). You also can use the distant and local points as accompanying points but usually just using the Ashi points are enough.

### <284> Wrist tenosynovitis, De Quervain's disease (1)

This is an inflammation of the synovial membrane. The patients experience the pain and have a difficulty in moving. Medical consultation is essential. There are infection and non-infection types. The main treatment idea is to regulate the Qi and blood on the local area and to promote the recovery. It is good to treat it in an occidental medicine and TCM way at the same time.

The main points : TB-5 ( Wai guan ), ST-41 ( Jie xi ), PC-3 ( Qu ze ), Ba xie ( Ex ), Shang ba xie ( Ex ), PC-7 ( Da ling ), GB-34 ( Yang ling quan ), Liv-3 ( Tai chong ), PC-6 ( Nei guan )

The accompanying points : GB-40 ( Qiu xu ), SP-6 ( San yin jiao ), SP-9 ( Yin ling quan ), TB-10 ( Tian jing ), Shi xuan ( Ex ) : bloodletting technique

The local and distant points are used to regulate the Qi and blood of the local area. Ba xie and Shang ba xie are the extra acupoints on the hands. They improve the local circulation and relieve the pain. Ba xie is a group of points at the sides of the fingers. Shang ba xie is slightly above the Ba xie on the dorsal side of hand. Ba xie, Shang ba xie can regulate the Qi and blood of the upper limbs. Shi xuan is the extra acupoints of the hands. The location is on the ends of the each finger. The acupoints on the ankle are used because the wrist corresponds to the ankle. The acupoints on the SP channel are used because they eliminate the dampness on the articulations. The bleeding method is used on Shi xuan. The strong manipulation is used.

### <285> Wrist tenosynovitis, De Quervain's disease (2)

This is an inflammation of the synovial membrane. The patients experience the pain and have a difficulty in moving. Medical consultation is essential. There are infection and non-infection types. The main treatment idea is to regulate the Qi and blood on the local area and to promote the recovery. It is good to treat it in an occidental medicine and TCM way at the same time.

The main points : GB-34 ( Yang ling quan ), Lu-9 ( Tai yuan ), Liv-3 ( Tai chong ), Lu-10 ( Yu ji ), GB-21 ( Jian jing ), LI-10 ( Shou san li ), Lu-7 ( Lie que ), LI-4 ( He gu ), Ashi
The accompanying points : GB-31 ( Feng shi ), Lu-5 ( Chi ze ), ST-36 ( Zu san li ), SP-9 ( Yin ling quan )

The local and distant points are used to relieve the pain and swelling. The strong manipulation is used. The moxibustion or intradermal needles can be used on the Ashi points

# | 24 |

# Kidneys and urination

**<286> Cystitis ( Inflammation of lower urinary tract or bladder )**

This is an infection at the lower urinary tract, or the urinary bladder. Medical consultation is essential. There are uncomplicated or complicated cases. Uncomplicated cystitis are about UTI in men or non- pregnant healthy women. The main treatment idea is to promote the urination by activating the kidneys, urinary bladder, lung, spleen and liver, and to eliminate the pathogens from the urinary tract. In chronic cases, strengthening the body to activate the immune system is necessary.

The main points : CV-3 ( Zhong ji ), CV-4 ( Guan yuan ), CV-2 ( Qu gu ), BL-32 ( Ci liao ), BL-23 ( Shen shu ), SP-9 ( Yin ling quan ), ST-29 ( Gui lai ), K-12 ( Da he ), Lu-5 ( Chi ze )

The accompanying points : CV-9 ( Shui fen ), LI-11 ( Qu chi ), ST-36 ( Zu san li ), LI-4 ( He gu ), K-10 ( Yin gu ), Liv-8 ( Qu quan ), BL-40 ( Wei zhong ), K-6 ( Zhao hai ), BL-60 ( Kun lun ), K-7 ( Fu liu ), BL-28 ( Pang guang shu )

K-7, K-10 and K-12 activate the kidneys. CV-3 promotes the urination and eliminates the pathogen from the urinary tract. BL:-24 and BL-28 eliminate the pathogen from the urinary tract and regulate the Qi and blood of the lower burner. ST-29 eliminates the pathogens from the urinary tract and regulates the Qi and blood of the lower burner. BL-23 activates the kidneys. BL-40 promotes the urination. BL-32 eliminates the pathogen and regulate the Qi and blood in the sacral region. CV-2 promotes the urination and eliminates the pathogen from the lower burner. Liv-8 nourishes the liver and eliminates the pathogens. BL-60 is the distant point. The strong manipulation is used for the acute case. The moxibustion is used for chronic cases.

### <287> Dysuria ( Painful urination )

This is not a disease but a symptom of painful urination or burning sensation in urination. Medical consultation is essential. Usually the urinary tract inflammation can cause dysuria. The pregnant women, diabetes or any problem of urinary bladder can cause dysuria. In TCM view, the burning sensation and painful urination is damp heat. The main treatment idea in TCM is to promote the urination and to eliminate the damp heat. SP, BL and Liv channels are important.

The main points : Lu-5 ( Chi ze ), BL-40 ( Wei zhong ) : bloodletting technique, ST-30 ( Qi chong ), BL-28 ( Pang guang shu ), CV-3 ( Zhong ji ), CV-4 ( Guan yuan ), SP-9 ( Yin ling quan )

The accompanying points : Liv-3 ( Tai chong ), K-7 ( Fu liu ), CV-9 ( Shui fen ), BL-64 ( Jing gu ), BL-33 ( Zhong liao ), BL-32 ( Ci liao ), CV-2 ( Qu gu ), Liv-8 ( Qu quan ), Long men ( Ex ), K-11 ( Heng gu )

BL-40 is for urination and to eliminate the blood stagnation. CV-3 and CV-2 promote urination and eliminate the damp heat. BL-28, BL-32 and BL-33 eliminate the pathogen from the lower burner. SP-6, Liv-8 and SP-9 eliminate the dampness. Long men is the extra acupoint for urinary problem. The location is at the lower edge of the pubic bone on the conception vessel (Ren mai). Long men has a very good effect on difficulty in urination. ST-30 and K-11 eliminate the pathogen from the lower burner and regulate the Qi and blood in urinary bladder. The strong manipulation is used for the main points in case of acute or excess cases. Soft manipulation is used for the chronic or deficiency cases. The prescription can be modified depending on the syndromes or patterns.

### <288> Enuresis ( Bed wetting, nocturnal enuresis, diurnal enuresis )

The symptoms are repeated wetting in the clothes, bed-wetting or wetting more than twice a week in three months. Medical consultation is essential. But this is not diagnosed unless the child is 5 years old or more than 5 years old. There are many different causes of enuresis but usually mental stress, urinary tract inflammation, small urinary bladder or developmental delays are the causes. In TCM view, this is the deficiency of spleen and kidneys. Most commonly the deficiency of Yang of spleen and kidneys are the main causes and the heat in the heart from mental stress can be the important cause. The mental stress may be the cause when the patients give too much stress to the child. The mental stress can generate the heat in the heart and liver Qi stagnation. The main treatment idea is to tonify the spleen and kidneys to control the urination.

The main points : CV-4 ( Guan yuan ), CV-3 ( Zhong ji ), GV-20 ( Bai hui ), Liv-8 ( Qu quan ), K-3 ( Tai xi ), BL-39 ( Wei yang ), Ht-8 ( Shao fu ), Liv-3 ( Tai chong ), CV-2 ( Qu gu )

The accompanying points : K-7 ( Fu liu ), SP-6 ( San yin jiao ), GV-4 ( Ming men ) : moxibustion can be used for cold syndrome, ST-36 ( Zu san li ), BL-32 ( Ci liao ), BL-64 ( Jing gu ), BL-40 ( Wei zhong )

ST-36 and K-3 tonify the spleen and kidneys. Ht-8 clears the heat in the heart and calm the mental stress or tension. CV-3 regulates the urination. Liv-3 relieves the mental stress from liver Qi stagnation.

BL-39 and BL-32 regulate the urination. CV-2 regulates the urination. SP-6 strengthens the kidneys, liver and spleen. Liv-8 regulates the urination. The middle level manipulation is used.

### <289> Frequent urination

This is a symptom that the patient pees more often than average (6~8 times a day). It's common in people older than 70, enlarged prostate or pregnant women. The most commonly seen cause is urinary tract infection. Medical consultation is essential. If there is urinary tract infection, it is necessary to treat the infection. The main treatment idea is to regulate and tonify the kidneys and spleen and to eliminate the infection. If there is mental stress, it is necessary to relieve the liver Qi stagnation and calm the heart.

The main points : Liv-8 ( Qu quan ), BL-32 ( Ci liao ), Liv-3 ( Tai chong ), BL-40 ( Wei zhong ), GV-20 ( Bai hui ), CV-9 ( Shui fen ), ST-28 ( Shui dao ), ST-36 ( Zu san li ), K-3 ( Tai xi )

The accompanying points : CV-4 ( Guan yuan ), GB-34 ( Yang ling quan ), BL-39 ( Wei yang ), BL-23 ( Shen shu ), K-7 ( Fu liu ), CV-3 ( Zhong ji ), CV-2 ( Qu gu ), BL-64 ( Jing gu )

If the cause is mental stress, add Yin tang ( Ex ), Ht-7 ( Shen men ), Liv-2 ( Xing jian ), LI-4 ( He gu ), PC-6 ( Nei guan )

Liv-3 regulates the liver and eliminates the mental stress from liver Qi stagnation. BL-64 regulates the urination. BL-40 regulates the urination and removes the blood stagnation. Liv-8 eliminates the dampness from the urinary tract. CV-2 and CV-3 regulate the urination and eliminate the pathogen from the urinary tract. BL-32 eliminates the pathogen from the lower burner. BL-23 tonifies the kidneys. GB-34 eliminates the dampness. Ht-7 and PC-6 are to calm the mind. The middle level manipulation is used. The moxibustion is used on the area of inferior abdomen or CV-2,3 for deficiency or chronic cases.

### <290> Glomerulonephritis, GN

This is inflammation and damage to the glomerulus of the kidneys. It can be acute or chronic. As a result, metabolic wastes are not filtered into the urine and can accumulate in the body. The patient can experience edema and fatigue. Medical consultation is essential. In TCM view the patient can experience the deficiency of kidneys, lung and heart. The main treatment idea is to eliminate the inflammation, to regulate and tonify the kidneys Yang in case of deficiency.

The main points : K-7 ( Fu liu ), ST-36 ( Zu san li ), K-10 ( Yin gu ), CV-4 ( Guan yuan ), BL-23 ( Shen shu ), GV-4 ( Ming men ), K-3 ( Tai xi ), BL-40 ( Wei zhong ), BL-22 ( San jiao shu ), SP-6 ( San yin jiao ), BL-52 ( Zhi shi ), CV-6 ( Qi hai )

The accompanying points :

If the heart is weak, add PC-6 ( Nei guan ), BL-15 ( Xin shu ), PC-4 ( Ji men ) or Ht-7 ( Shen men )

if the quantity of urine decreases, add SP-9 ( Yin ling quan ), BL-26 ( Guan yuan shu ), BL-39 ( Wei yang ).

If the breath is short, add BL-13 ( Fei shu ), BL-17 ( Ge shu ), SP-4 ( Gong sun ), GV-12 ( Shen zhu ).

BL-23 tonifies the kidneys. GV-4 warms the kidneys Yang. BL-52 nourishes the kidneys essence. BL-22 regulates the TB. CV-6, CV-4 and SP-6 strengthen the kidneys and liver, and eliminate the dampness from the lower burner. The accompanying points can be added depending on the symptoms. The strong manipulation is used for acute cases. Moxibustion is used for chronic cases.

### <291> Hematuria ( Presence of blood in urine )

There are many causes of hematuria and if any cause is known, it is necessary to treat that cause. Medical consultation is essential. Here the prescription is focused on the stopping the bleeding. In TCM view, mainly the damp heat on the lower burner, deficiency of spleen Qi or blood stagnation are the main pathological patterns. The main treatment idea is to eliminate the damp heat, tonify the spleen or remove the blood stagnation.

The main points : Long men ( Ex ), SP-6 ( San yin jiao ), SP-10 ( Xue hai ), BL-17 ( Ge shu ), GB-34 ( Yang ling quan ), ST-27 ( Da ju ), SP-1 ( Yin bai ), CV-3 ( Zhong ji ), BL-26 ( Guan yuan shu ), SP-9 ( Yin ling quan ), BL-23 ( Shen shu )

The accompanying points : ST-30 ( Qi chong ), LI-11 ( Qu chi ), BL-31 ( Shang liao ), BL-32 ( Ci liao ), ST-24 ( Huo rou men ), LI-4 ( He gu ), K-9 ( Zhu bin ), ST-36 ( Zu san li ), BL-19 ( Dan shu ), CV-2 ( Qu gu )

ST-36 tonifies the spleen Qi and eliminates the dampness. In case of damp heat or excess syndrome, you need to use reducing methods on ST-36 to eliminate the dampness. GB-34 eliminates the dampness. CV-3 and CV-2 eliminate the damp heat from the lower burner. SP-6 and SP-9 eliminate the damp heat. Long men is the extra acupoint to eliminate the dampness and promote the urination. The location of Long men is at the lower border of the pubic bone on the conception vessel ( Ren mai ). The strong manipulation is used. The medical examination is necessary to prevent the delay of treatment of severe causes like cancer.

### <292> Kidneys stone ( Renal calculi, Nephrolithiasis, Urolithiasis )

The main causes are genetic, wrong diet ( for example, too much taking spinach and calcium together can form stone easily ) or too much taking meat products etc. Medical consultation is essential. In TCM view stones in the body are damp heat. If the stones are too big, medical surgery is considered but if the stones are not big, acupuncture and TCM herbal medicine treatment can be used. The main treatment idea is to promote the urination and eliminate the damp heat.

The main points : BL-40 ( Wei zhong ), CV-3 ( Zhong ji ), SP-6 ( San yin jiao ), K-16 ( Huang shu ), GB-25 ( Jing men ), SP-9 ( Yin ling quan ), BL-22 ( San jiao shu ), CV-2 ( Qu gu ), K-10 ( Yin gu ), BL-24 ( Qi hai shu ), GB-26 ( Dai mai ), BL-23 ( Shen shu )

The accompanying points : LI-11 ( Qu chi ), ST-40 ( Feng long ), BL-60 ( Kun lun ), SP-15 ( Da heng ), K-3 ( Tai xi ), BL-64 ( Jing gu ), SP-14 ( Fu jie ), SP-10 ( Xue hai ), ST-36 ( Zu san li )

The main points are to promote the urination and eliminate the damp heat. The accompanying points are used to relieve the pain. Sometimes, the stone is removed by acupuncture in case the stone is not that big. TCM Herbal medicine is used too. The strong manipulation is used. If the stone is too big, medical surgery is necessary.

### <293> Nephrosis ( Nephrotic syndrome )

The causes are damages at the clusters of small vessels of kidneys. That part filters waste and excess water. Medical consultation is essential. The patient experiences swelling in feet or ankles. And it threatens the life when becomes severe. In TCM view, it is the deficiency of Kidneys Yang.

The main points : TB-3 ( Zhong zhu ), GV-4 ( Ming men ), CV-9( Shui fen ), CV-4 ( Guan yuan ), K-7 ( Fu liu ), BL-52 ( Zhi shi ), BL-23 ( Shen shu )

The accompanying points : ST-36 ( Zu san li ), GV-3 ( Yao yang guan ), SP-6 ( San yin jiao ), CV-6 ( Qi hai ), SI-3 ( Hou xi ), BL-22 ( San jiao shu ), K-16 ( Huang shu ), LI-11 ( Qu chi )

The main points and accompanying points are to tonify the kidneys Yang, Qi and regulate the kidneys function. The long term treatment is necessary with moxibustion. The middle level manipulation of needles can be used.

### <294> Pyelitis ( Pyelonephritis )

This is a bacterial infection of the renal pelvis. The main cause is urinary tract infection or a bladder infection. Medical consultation is essential. If a lower urinary tract infection is not properly treated, the bacteria can infect the renal pelvis. Kidneys stones or ureteral stones are also responsible for Pyelitis. In occidental medicine, it is treated with antibiotics. The main treatment idea in TCM is to eliminate the damp heat. In chronic case, tonifying method is used at the same time.

The main points : LI-11 ( Qu chi ), BL-64 ( Jing gu ), GB-26 ( Dai mai ), BL-22 ( San jiao shu ), BL-23 ( Shen shu ), LI-4 ( He gu ), K-16 ( Huang shu ), CV-4 ( Guan yuan )

The accompanying points : SP-6 ( San yin jiao ), BL-40 ( Wei zhong ), GV-4 ( Ming men ), K-3 ( Tai xi ), ST-24 ( Huo rou men ), BL-52 ( Zhi shi ), K-7 ( Fu liu )

The main points and the accompanying points are to eliminate the damp heat and eliminate the inflammation. K-3, BL-52 and BL-23 tonify the kidneys for deficiency case and regulate the kidneys function for acute and excess cases. CV-4 and K-7 activate the Kidneys yang for deficiency case and regulate the kidneys function for acute and excess cases. The strong manipulation is used without leaving the needles for acute cases and excess syndromes. The moxibustion is used for chronic or deficiency cases.

### <295> Renal atrophy

The main causes of renal atrophy are blocked urinary tract, kidneys stones or long term kidneys infection. Medical consultation is essential. In TCM, the main treatment idea is to tonify kidneys, regulate the blood circulation in kidneys, recover the urinary tract and eliminate the kidneys stones. The additional treatment can be done following the symptoms.

The main points : SP-6 ( San yin jiao ), CV-4 ( Guan yuan ), K-7 ( Fu liu ), K-6 ( Zhao hai ), BL-23 ( Shen shu ), K-1 ( Yong quan ), ST-36 ( Zu san li ), GB-21 ( Jian jing ), GB-20 ( Feng chi )

The accompanying points :

In case of frequent urination at night, add BL-64 ( Jing gu ), GV-20 ( Bai hui ), CV-3 ( Zhong ji )

In case of ear ringing, add SI-4 ( Wan gu ), TB-3 ( Zhong zhu ), GB-41 ( Zu lin qi ), TB-21 ( Er men ).

In case of dizziness and insomnia, add GV-20 ( Bai hui ), GV-12 ( Shen zhu ), BL-14 ( Jue yin shu ), BL-12 ( Feng men ), GB-20 ( Feng chi )

The main points tonify and regulate the functions of kidneys and promote the blood circulation in kidneys. GB-20 relieves the dizziness from renal atrophy. CV-4 and K-7 tonify the kidneys. Depending on the symptoms the proper modification of addition of points are possible. The moxibustion is used. The soft manipulation of needles can be used.

### <296> Renal tuberculosis ( Renal TB )

The main cause is Mycobacterium tuberculosis and is the most common form. Medical consultation is essential. Renal TB is more likely to develop with pulmonary tuberculosis. In main treatment idea is to tonify kidneys and eliminate the pathological heat.

The main points : K-16 ( Huang shu ), Lu-7 ( Lie que ), BL-23 ( Shen shu ), CV-12 ( Zhong wan ), CV-3 ( Zhong ji ), K-3 ( Tai xi ), SP-6 ( San yin jiao )

The accompanying points : Lu-10 ( Yu ji ), K-2 ( Ran gu ), BL-13 ( Fei shu ), BL-20 ( Pi shu ), LI-11 ( Qu chi ), Lu-5 ( Chi ze ), K-7 ( Fu liu ), BL-52 ( Zhi shi )

In case of stranguria, add SP-6 ( San yin jiao ), SP-9 ( Yin ling quan ), BL-64 ( Jing gu ), ST-30 ( Qi chong ), CV-9 ( Shui fen )

K-3, BL-23, K-16 and K-9 nourish the kidneys. CV-3 promotes the urination and eliminates the dampness. Lu-5 activates the lung to help the kidneys function and to eliminate the lung TB. The method of tonifying lung and spleen are used to help the kidneys function. In case of stranguria, the accompanying points can be added. The moxibustion is used on the main points. In case of high fever, the needles are used.

### <297> Uremia ( Urine poisoning )

This is about high levels of urea in the blood. This can be an important indicator of renal failure. Medical consultation is essential. If it becomes severe, it can be life threatening. The symptoms are fatigue, weakness, vomiting, nausea, loss of appetite, tremor, muscle atrophy, mental problem, superficial breathing etc. Usually uremia is the result of renal failure and can lead to coma and death. The emergency treatment in medical hospital is necessary. TCM treatment can be used at the same time to increase the therapeutic effects. This is a kind of collapse of Qi and Yang in TCM view that makes the coma and total deficiency.

The main points : CV-4 ( Guan yuan ), K-2 ( Ran gu ), CV-2 ( Qu gu ), GV-14 ( Da zhui ), LI-11 ( Qu chi ), LI-4 ( He gu ), Liv-3 ( Tai chong )

The accompanying points : SP-6 ( San yin jiao ), GV-20 ( Bai hui ), K-1 ( Yong quan ), Liv-2 ( Xing jian )

The main points and the accompanying points open the orifice to awaken the consciousness and tonify the Qi and Yang. The medical treatment is necessary. The moxibustion is used. Treatment of the cause is important.

### <298> Urethritis ( Inflammation of urethra )

This is a lower urinary tract infection. This disease has close association with STIs, sexually transmitted infections. Medical consultation is essential. The main causes are bacteria and viruses. The main symptom is painful urination. In TCM view, this is damp heat in the lower burner. The main treatment idea is to clear the damp heat.

The main points : K-6 ( Zhao hai ), CV-2 ( Qu gu ), SP-9 ( Yin ling quan ), BL-64 ( Jing gu ), BL-40 ( Wei zhong ), CV-3 ( Zhong ji ), SP-6 ( San yin jiao ), Liv-8 ( Qu quan ), Long men ( Ex ), BL-32 ( Ci liao )

The accompanying points : BL-23 ( Shen shu ), K-12 ( Da he ), GV-4 ( Ming men ) : for cold syndrome, Liv-3 ( Tai chong ), Liv-2 ( Xing jian ), ST-30 ( Qi chong ), Liv-9 ( Yin bao )

Long men is the extra acupoint to eliminate the dampness and to promote the urination. The location is at the lower border of the pubic bone at the CV channel. The main points and the accompanying points are to eliminate the damp heat in the urinary tract and to promote the urination. The strong manipulation is used without leaving the needles for acute cases. The moxibustion is used for chronic or deficiency cases.

### <299> Urinary incontinence

This is about leaking urine by accident. This is common in old age. Medical consultation is essential. The causes are not clearly known but probably too much intake of alcohol or caffeine are related with urinary incontinence. In TCM view, this is deficiency of Qi in spleen and kidneys. Lung, spleen, kidneys and liver are related. The main treatment idea is to tonify Qi in spleen and kidneys and to activate the lung to regulate the urination.

The main points : ST-36 ( Zu san li ), CV-4 ( Guan yuan ), GV-20 ( Bai hui ), CV-3 ( Zhong ji ), BL-32 ( Ci liao ), K-7 ( Fu liu ), BL-39 ( Wei yang ), Lu-7 ( Lie que ), Liv-3 ( Tai chong )

The accompanying points : SP-9 ( Yin ling quan ), BL-23 ( Shen shu ), BL-60 ( Kun lun ), SP-6 ( San yin jiao ), GV-4 ( Ming men ), K-6 ( Zhao hai ), CV-2 ( Qu gu ), Liv-8 ( Qu quan )

The main points and the accompanying points are to regulate the urination, strengthen the spleen and kidneys and activate the lung function. GV-20 hold the Qi not to fall. The soft manipulation is used. Moxibustion can used.

**<300> Urinary retention, Ischuria**

This is a symptom that the patient is not able to empty all urine from the bladder. Medical consultation is essential. The main causes are obstruction or narrowing around the bladder, or when muscles around the bladder are weak. And the other causes are constipation, tumor, some medications or being dehydrated. If any causes are known, it is necessary to treat that cause. Here this prescription is focused on the symptom itself. In TCM view, this is the deficiency of spleen, kidneys and lung. The main treatment idea is to tonify spleen, kidneys and lung to promote the urination and regulate the urination.

The main points : CV-4 ( Guan yuan ), SP-6 ( San yin jiao ), K-7 ( Fu liu ), Long men ( Ex ), SP-9 ( Yin ling quan ), CV-3 ( Zhong ji ), Liv-2 ( Xing jian ), Lu-7 ( Lie que )

The accompanying points : BL-32 ( Ci liao ), ST-36 ( Zu san li ), BL-13 ( Fei shu ), BL-28 ( Pang guang shu ), BL-23 ( Shen shu ), GV-4 ( Ming men ), BL-40 ( Wei zhong )

Liv-2 relieves the tension or contraction of the muscles around the bladder. BL-40 promotes the urination. CV-3 promotes the urination. Long men is the extra acupoint for urination and the location is at the lower border of the pubic bone at the CV channel. SP-9 promotes urination. BL-23 tonifies kidneys. BL-28 activates the movement of urinary bladder. SP-6 tonifies spleen. The strong manipulation is used.

# | 25 |

# Discussion about acupuncture for cancer

### <300> Cancer ( Discussion )

There are numerous types of cancer, and it is not easy to provide specific acupuncture prescriptions in this context. All cancer patients must seek medical consultation. To ensure safe and effective acupuncture practice, one can refer to the general Traditional Chinese Medicine (TCM) acupuncture prescription guidelines while considering necessary precautions. For all cancer cases, medical consultation and treatment are essential. In cancer treatment, acupuncture cannot replace medical treatment. In China, a combination of Western medical treatment and traditional Chinese herbal medicine is commonly used.

Acupuncture offers several merits when integrated into the care of cancer patients. Depending on the patient's condition, acupuncture and massage can be beneficial during specific phases of their cancer. In cases where cancer patients have undergone curative surgery and are in the recovery phase, Acupuncture and massage can play a role in their rehabilitation. These therapies primarily focus on improving blood circulation, resolving blood stasis, reducing fatigue, and relaxing muscle tension. Moreover, it aids in psychological adjustment, contributing to the overall mental and physical well-being of the patient.

However, when dealing with cancer patients in an active tumor state, great caution is essential, and thorough knowledge of the patient's medical history is crucial. For instance, if a cancer patient has bone metastases, acupuncture or massage on those bones can increase the risk of pathological bone fractures. Additionally, acupuncture and massage on visible lymph node enlargement, subcutaneous nodules on the patient's body or on the tumor can increase the possibility of metastasis, potentially promoting tumor spread, especially via needle-induced pathways. Some patients may even develop infections due to acupuncture because of low immune functions of the cancer patients, which could lead to treatment delays. Therefore, it is generally not advisable for patients with active tumors to undergo these therapies.

Cancer patients often experience a heightened tendency for blood clotting, resulting in a sixfold higher risk of venous thromboembolism (VTE) compared to non-cancer patients, particularly in the form of deep vein thrombosis (DVT) in the lower limbs. DVT itself is not typically alarming, but if a clot dislodges, it can lead to severe complications such as heart attacks, pulmonary embolisms, or strokes. Massaging the lower limbs without prior knowledge of the presence of deep vein thrombosis can trigger clot dislodgment, resulting in serious issues. Hence, when family members provide leg massages to late-stage cancer patients, confirming the absence of deep vein thrombosis is imperative, typically through vascular ultrasound imaging. Furthermore, patients with a tendency to bleed may be at risk of bleeding due to mechanical stimulation during acupuncture and massage.

Application of acupuncture should be carried out with great care and consideration of the patient's specific medical condition and history. Patients and their families should consult with healthcare professionals to ensure that acupuncture treatments are safe and appropriate for their individual needs.

# | 26 |

# Bibliography

1. Giovanni Maciocia. The foundations of Chinese Medicine. 3rd Edition, Elsevier, 2015.
2. Giovanni Maciocia. The practice of Chinese Medicine. 2nd Edition, Elsevier, 2008.
3. Unschuld P. Ling Shu. University of California Press, USA, 2016.
4. Lee Hyen Soon, Rodem Namu. Introduction to Acupuncture (Chimguhakgyeron), South Korea, 2007.
5. The complete Art of Acupuncture (Zhen Jiu Da Cheng ), Yang Ji Zhou ( Ming dynasty in China ), Traditional Chinese Medicine Ancient Texts Publishing House ( Zhong Yi Gu Ji Chu Ban She ), China, 1998
6. Expounding on the fourteen channels ( Shi Si Jing Fa Hui ). Hua Shou ( Yuan dynasty in China ), Henan Science and Technology press ( He Nan Ke Xue Ji Shu Chu Ban She ), China, 2014
7. Acupuncture and Moxibustion Therapy ( Zhen Jiu Zhi Liao Xue ), Gao Shu Zhong, Yang Ji Guo, Jia Guo Yan, Shanghai Science and Technology892nd Press ( Shang hai ke xue ji shu chu ban she ), China, 2018
8. Acupuncture and Moxibustion Studies ( Zhen Jiu Xue ), Yan Ping, Science Press ( Ke Xue Chu Ban She ), China, 2004
9. Atlas of Extra Acupoints in Acupuncture and Moxibustion, Hao Jin Kai, People's Military Medical Press ( Ren Min Jun Yi Chu Ban She ), China, 2011

10. Pernkopf Anatomy, Werner Platzer, Urban & Schwarzenberg; Germany, 1989

11. The Complete Dictionary of Ailments and Diseases, Jacques Martel, New Leaf Distributing, 2012

12. The Encyclopedia of Ailments and Diseases, Jacques Martel, Findhorn Press, 2nd Edition, 2020

13. SNUH Manual of Medicine, Department of Internal Medicine, Seoul National University, College of Medicine, 6th Edition, South Korea, 2022

| 27 |

# INDEX

: Names of diseases or health conditions - Index number

Abdominal pain - 145

Accumulation in heart ( Xin ji ) - five accumulation ( Wu ji ) (1) - 146

Accumulation in kidneys ( Shen ji ) - five accumulation ( Wu ji ) (2) - 147

Accumulation in liver ( Gan ji ) - five accumulation ( Wu ji ) (3) - 148

Accumulation in lungs ( Fei ji ) - five accumulation ( Wu ji ) (4) - 149

Accumulation in spleen ( Pi ji ) - five accumulation ( Wu ji ) (5) - 150

Achilles tendinitis - 237

Acute backpain (1) - 238

Acute backpain (2) - 239

Acute backpain (3) - 240

Addison's disease, Chronic adrenal insufficiency - 151

Adnexitis, inflammation of the uterine appendages - 112

Agalactia, Low breast milk supply - 113

Alopecia Areata ( Patchy hair loss ) - 33

Amenorrhea (1) - 114

Amenorrhea (2) - 115

Amyotrophic lateral sclerosis (ALS), Lou Gehrig's disease - 241

Anemia - 152
Angina pectoris - 140
Ankle joint pain - 242
Ankylosing spondylitis - 243
Appendicitis - 38
Arteriosclerosis - 153
Ascites - 154
Auditory vertigo, Meniere syndrome - 69
Bacillary dysentery - 39
Bad breath ( halitosis ) - 155
Benign prostatic hyperplasia - 194
Beriberi, thiamine deficiency - 156
Bipolar disorder, manic-depressive disorder - 1
Bronchial asthma - 227
Bronchiectasis - 228
Bronchitis - 229
Bruise, contusion - 244
Cancer (Discussion) - 301
Cardiac asthma - 230
Cardiac neurosis - 2
Carsickness, seasickness or airsickness ( motion sickness ) - 157
Cataract - 90
Cerebral anemia - 3
Cerebral congestion - 4
Chest pain - 158
Cholecystitis, inflammation of gall bladder - 189
Cholelithiasis, gall stone - 190
Chronic backpain - 245
Cirrhosis - 191
Cold (1) - 102
Cold (2) heat type with unclear consciousness - 103
Colitis (1) - 40
Colitis (2) acute case - 41
Colitis (3) chronic case - 42

Conjunctivitis - 91
Constipation - 43
Corn, Clavus - 34
Cough - 231
Cramp in legs, cramp in gastrocnemius - 246
CVA, brain stroke – aphasia - 6
CVA, brain stroke - blocking syndrome - 7
CVA, brain stroke - facial paralysis - 8
CVA, brain stroke - paralysis of lower limbs - 9
CVA, brain stroke - paralysis of upper limbs - 10
CVA, brain stroke – prevention - 11
CVA, brain stroke – prodrome - 12
CVA, brain stroke - seven points - 5
CVA, brain stroke - syndrome of collapse - 13
Cystitis (Inflammation of lower urinary tract or bladder) - 286
Deaf-mutism, surdimutism - 70
Deafness (1) - sequelae of a disease - 71
Deafness (2) - sequelae of a disease - 72
Degenerative arthritis of knee - 247
Dentoalveolar abscess – 30
Depression - 29
Diabetes mellitus, syndrome of consumptive thirst - 159
Diarrhea (1) - 44
Diarrhea (2) - 45
Diarrhea (3) - with colic - 46
Difficulty in breathing - 232
Drowning - 160
Duodenal ulcer - 47
Dysfunctional uterine bleeding (DUB) - 116
Dysuria (Painful urination) - 287
Ear pain - 73
Edema - 161
Electric ophthalmia, Arc flash ophthalmitis - 92
Electric shock - 162

Emphysema - 233
Endocarditis - 141
Enuresis (Bed wetting, nocturnal enuresis, diurnal enuresis) - 288
Epilepsy (1) - 14
Epilepsy (2) - 15
Epilepsy (3) - 16
Epistaxis - 74
EPS ( Extrapyramidal symptoms ) - 17
Erectile dysfunction (1) - 195
Erectile dysfunction (2) - 196
Esophageal stenosis - 75
Esophagus spasms - 76
Excessive menstruation - 117
Excessive vaginal discharge - 118
Eye pain - 93
Facial nerve paralysis - 203
Facial spasm - 204
Feel cold - 163
Female infertility - 119
Fever - 104
Fibromyalgia syndrome (FMS) - 248
Frequent urination - 289
Frostbite - 164
Frozen shoulder (Adhesive capsulitis) - 249
Gastric atony - 48
Gastric hyperacidity - 49
Gastritis - 50
Gastroptosis - 51
Gingivitis - 31
Glaucoma - 94
Glomerulonephritis (GN) - 290
Goiter - 77
Gout - 165
Headache - frontal area - 134

Headache – general - 135
Heart pain - 142
Hematuria (Presence of blood in urine) - 291
Hemoptysis - 166
Hemorrhoids - 52
Hepatitis - 192
Hiccup - 53
Hives, Urticaria - 35
Hypertension - mild case - 167
Hypertension - severe case - 168
Hyperthyroidism - 169
Hypochlorhydria - 54
Hypotension - 170
Hysteria (1) - 18
Hysteria (2) - 19
Indigestion (1) - diarrhea, fever, vomiting - 55
Indigestion (2) - stagnation of food - 56
Infantile nearsightedness ( Myopia ) - 211
Influenza, the flu (1) - 105
Influenza, the flu (2) - 106
Insomnia - 20
Intercostal neuralgia - 205
Intestinal bleeding - 57
Intestinal obstruction, ileus - 58
Intestinal stenosis, enterostenosis - 59
Intestinal tuberculosis - 60
Jaundice - 193
Kidney stone (Renal calculi, Nephrolithiasis, Urolithiasis) - 292
Knee joint pain - 250
Loss of appetite - 61
Malaria - 107
Male infertility - 197
Malpresentation or fetal malposition - 120
Mastitis - 121

Menopause disorder - 122
Menstrual irregularity - 123
Menstrual pain - 124
Migraine - 136
Multiple sclerosis - lower limbs - 206
Multiple sclerosis - upper limbs - 207
Mumps, epidemic parotitis - 108
Myasthenia Gravis - 251
Myelitis - 208
Nausea and vomiting (1) - 62
Nausea and vomiting (2) - 63
Nephrosis (Nephrotic syndrome) - 293
Neurasthenia - 21
Neurosis - OCD, Phobia, Anxiety disorder - 22
Night blindness, Nyctalopia - 95
Night crying of babies - 23
Nocturnal emission - 198
Nocturnal sweating ( night sweats ) - 171
Obesity - 172
Occipital headache - 137
Occipital neuralgia - 138
Ocular fatigue, Asthenopia - 96
Olfactory disorder, dysosmia - 78
Oligomenorrhea, hypomenorrhea, insufficient menstruation - 125
Orchitis - 199
Otitis media - CSOM ( Chronic suppurative otitis media ) - 80
Otitis media - OME ( Otitis media with effusion ) - 79
Painless or easy delivery - 126
Palpitations - 143
Pancreatitis - 173
Parkinson's disease - 24
Pediatric acute seizure - 212
Pediatric asthma - 213
Pediatric constitutional weakness - 214

Pediatric diarrhea - 215
Pediatric febrile convulsion - 216
Pediatric functional dyspepsia ( difficulty in digestion ) - 217
Pediatric night astonishment - 218
Pediatric non febrile convulsion - 219
Pediatric stomatitis - 220
Pediatric vomiting - 221
Peritonitis - 174
Pertussis (Whooping cough, 100 days cough) - 234
Pharyngitis, sore throat - 81
Physical weakness - 175
Pleurisy - 176
Pneumonia - 235
Poliomyelitis (initial stage)-abdominal muscles - 222
Poliomyelitis (initial stage)-facial muscles - 226
Poliomyelitis (initial stage)-lower limbs - 223
Poliomyelitis (initial stage)-neck - 224
Poliomyelitis (initial stage)-upper limbs - 225
Postpartum hemorrhage - 127
Premature ejaculation - 200
Presbyopia, Eyesight of the aged - 97
Prolapse of anus - 64
Prostatitis - 201
Pruritus, itching - 36
Ptosis, drooping of the upper eyelids - 98
Pulmonary tuberculosis - 236
Pyelitis (Pyelonephritis) - 294
Raynaud disease - 252
Renal atrophy - 295
Renal tuberculosis (Renal TB) - 296
Retroverted uterus - 128
Rheumatoid arthritis (RA)-elbows - 255
Rheumatoid arthritis (RA)-finger - 256
Rheumatoid arthritis (RA)-hip joint - 253

Rheumatoid arthritis (RA)-knee - 257
Rheumatoid arthritis (RA)-shoulder pain - 254
Rheumatoid inflammation of ankle joint - 258
Rheumatoid pain of muscles - 259
Rheumatoid temporomandibular disorder - 260
Rhinitis by common cold - 82
Runny nose - 83
Schizophrenia (1) - 25
Schizophrenia (2) - 26
Sciatica - 209
Scrofula - 177
Sexual insensitivity, frigidity - 129
Sexual insensitivity, frigidity - 202
Shingles, Herpes Zoster (1) - on the face - 109
Shingles, Herpes Zoster (2) - on the chest, abdomen, lateral sides - 110
Shoulder and arm pain - 261
Shoulder joint pain - 262
Sinusitis - 84
Spasm of eyelid, Blepharospasm - 99
Sprain - 263
Sprain of elbow or knee joints (1) - 264
Sprain of elbow or knee joints (2) - 265
Sprain of elbow or knee joints (3) - 266
Sprain of elbow or knee joints (4) - 267
Sprain of elbow or knee joints (5) - 268
Sprain of elbow or knee joints (6) - 269
Sprain of wrist or ankle (1) - 270
Sprain of wrist or ankle (2) - 271
Sprain of wrist or ankle (3) - 272
Sprain of wrist or ankle (4) - 273
Sprain of wrist or ankle (5) - 274
Sprain of wrist or ankle (6) - 275
Stiff neck - 276

Stomach ache - acute case - 65
Stomach cancer - 66
Stomach spasm, gastrospasm - 67
Stomach ulcer - 68
Stomatitis - 178
Stuffy nose - 85
Stupefaction (1) - blocking syndrome - 179
Stupefaction (2) - collapsing syndrome - 180
Stye - 100
Sunstroke, heliosis (1) - 181
Sunstroke, heliosis (2) - 182
Suppurative arthritis of knee (Septic arthritis of knee) - 277
Suppurative inflammation of ankle joint (Septic arthritis of ankle joint) - 276
Sydenham's chorea (SC) - 27
Syncope, faint - 183
Tennis elbow (Lateral epicondylitis) - 279
Tenosynovitis of index finger - 280
Tetanus, lockjaw - 111
Thumb tenosynovitis - 281
Tinnitus - deficiency of Kidneys - 86
Tinnitus - Liver fire - 87
Tinnitus – nervousness - 88
Tonsilitis - 89
Toothache - 32
Total exhaustion (1) - 184
Total exhaustion (2) - 185
Trigeminal neuralgia - 210
Tympanites - 186
Upper arm pain - 282
Uremia (Urine poisoning) - 297
Urethritis (Inflammation of urethra) - 298
Urinary incontinence - 299
Urinary retention, Ischuria - 300

Uterine cancer - 130
Uterine fibroids ( Leiomyomas, Myomas ) - 131
Uterine prolapse - 132
Valvular heart disease - 144
Vertex headache - 139
Vertigo - 187
Vomiting blood, hematemesis - 188
Vomiting with pregnancy ( Morning sickness ) - 133
Warts - 37
Water eyes ( excessive tearing ), Epiphora - 101
Wrist ganglion or ankle ganglion (Ganglion cysts) - 283
Wrist tenosynovitis, De Quervain's disease (1) - 284
Wrist tenosynovitis, De Quervain's disease (1) - 285
Writer's cramp, graphospasm – 28

www.ingramcontent.com/pod-product-compliance
Lightning Source LLC
LaVergne TN
LVHW040136080526
838202LV00042B/2921